Clinics, Contraception, and Communication

Evaluation Studies of Family Planning Programs
in Four Latin American Countries

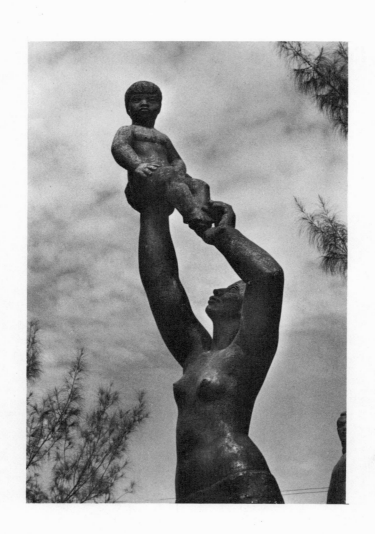

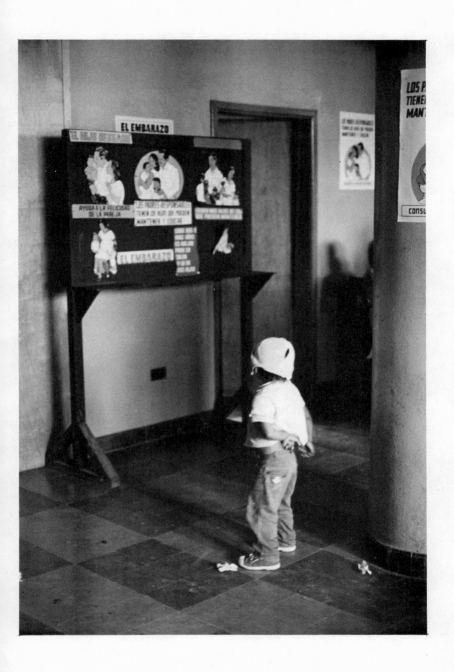

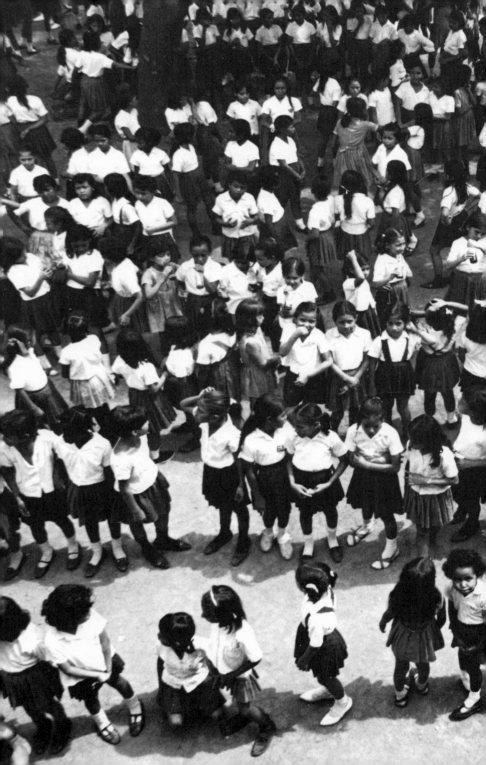

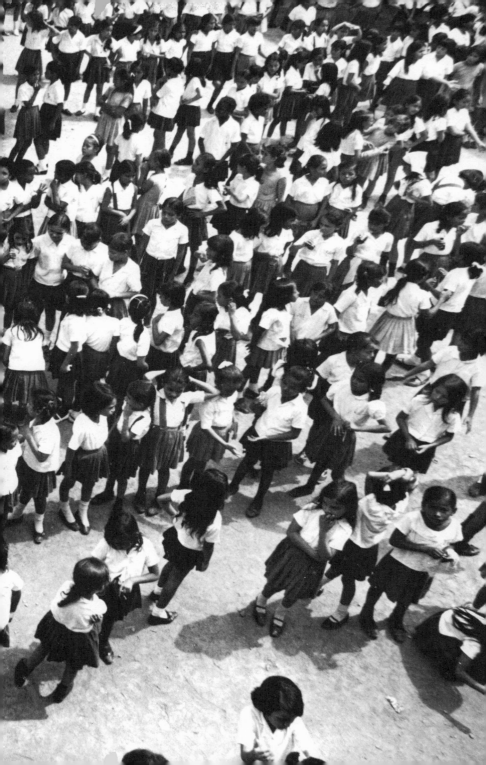

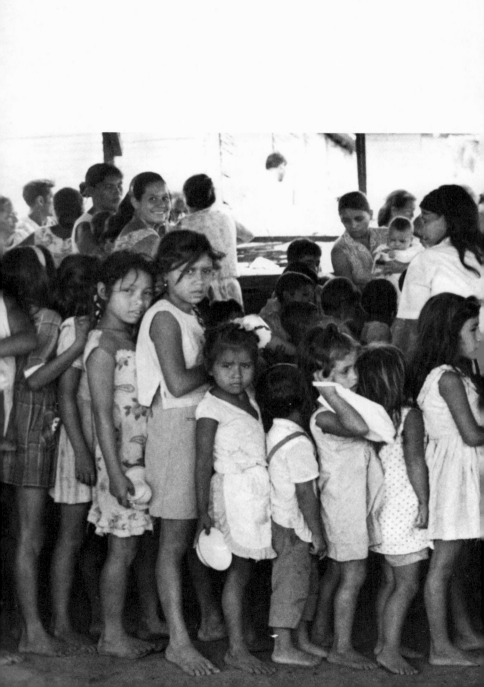

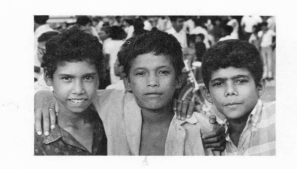

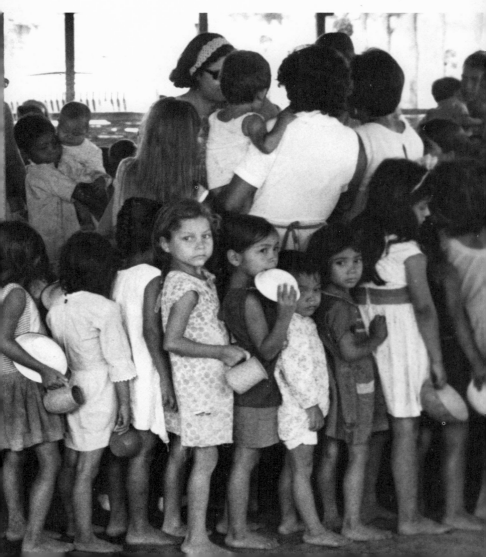

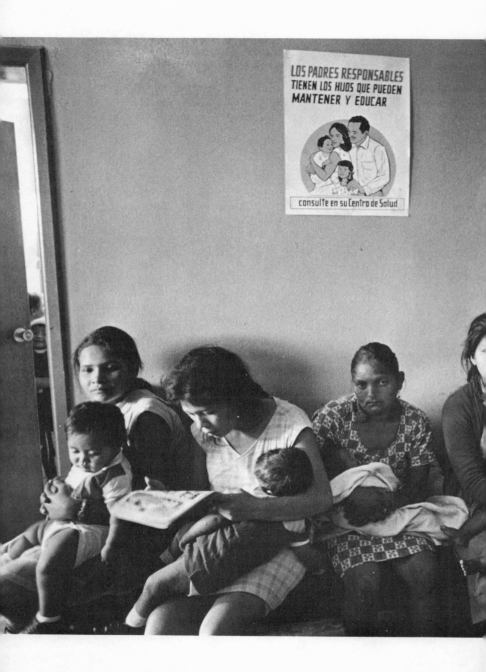

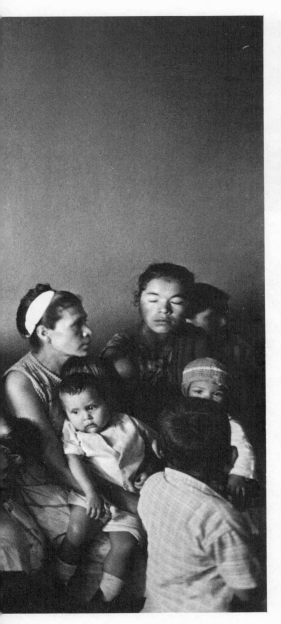
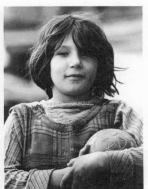

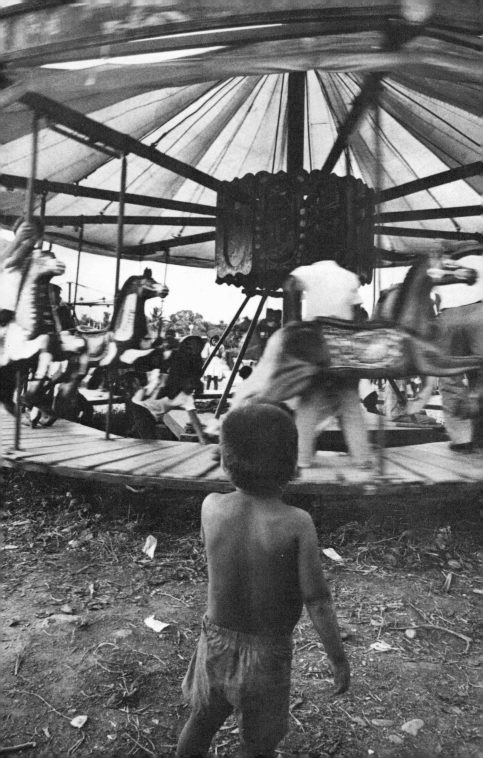

Clinics, Contraception, and Communication

Evaluation Studies of Family Planning Programs
in Four Latin American Countries

J. Mayone Stycos

with Alan B. Keller, Parker G. Marden, Anthony Marino,
Axel I. Mundigo, and Alan B. Simmons

New York
APPLETON-CENTURY-CROFTS
Educational Division
MEREDITH CORPORATION

ACC Population and Demography Series, Edited by J. Mayone Stycos

Published in cooperation with the International Population Program, Cornell Univer-sity, in association with the International Planned Parenthood Federation, Western Hemisphere.

Photographs by J. Mayone Stycos

Edited by Frances Benson and Barbara A. Stevens
Designed by David May

PRINTED IN THE UNITED STATES OF AMERICA

C-390-85609-6

Contents

Acknowledgments

Each of the five research projects described in this monograph was conceived and designed by an International Population Program collaborator and myself. Following each project design, the collaborator took over responsibility for the field work and analysis, and only following submission of a first draft report was my role again of any consequence, in most instances. In the case where I have assumed joint authorship with my colleague Professor Marden, I wrote about one-half of the report. In the Dominican study, Dr. Alan Simmons played an important part in the design.

As to the financing of these projects, we are pleased to acknowledge the assistance of the Population Council for the research reported in Chapters II and V, and the Agency for International Development (Honduran Mission) for the research in Chapters III and IV. The Population Council also supported the research reported in Chapter VI by a grant to the Dominican National Population and Family Council; as did the International Planned Parenthood Federation by a grant to the Dominican Association for Family Welfare.

Research in the field was usually carried out in collaboration with a local organization. In Honduras we owe special thanks to the Ministry of Health and its Maternal and Child Health Program for lending us essential services. Dr. Antonio Peraza, minister of health, and Dr. Danilo Velásquez were especially helpful. The cooperation and the contribution of office and meeting space by the Honduran Family Planning Association through its executive secretary, Lic. Alejandro Flores, deserve special acknowledgment.

In Colombia, the project was carried out jointly with the Population Division of the Colombian Association of Medical Schools. Its director, Dr. Guillermo Lopez, and its research director, Dr. Alcides Estrada, were generous with time, space, and general assistance in the field. Dr. Ramiro Cardona, director of Socio-Demographic Studies, and his staff assumed major responsibility for sampling and for interviewer recruitment and supervision. In addition, PROFAMILIA, the private family planning association, gave us free access to their files and generous support during the field operations. Dr. Fernando Tamayo and Dr. Gonzalo Echeverry were helpful at all crucial points of the research.

In Mexico, the research was carried out under the auspices of the Fundación para Estudios de la Población, where the administrative support of Lic. Gerardo Cornejo and the technical collaboration of Lic. Aurora Rabago and Lic. José Morelos were especially helpful. Dr. Sergio Correu, medical director of the Fundación, served as consultant.

In the Dominican Republic, the research was conducted under the joint auspices of the Consejo Nacional de Población y Familia and the Asociación Dominicana Pro Bienestar de la Familia. Their respective directors, Lic. Manuel Rodriguez Casado and Dr. Orestes Cucurullo, were particularly instrumental in all stages of the study. Also, special mention should be made of the office space, other facilities, and interviewers made available to us by the Centro de Investigación, under the direction of Ing. Ezequiel García, of Pedro Henríquez Ureña National University.

The publication assistance of the International Planned Parenthood Federation, Western Hemisphere, is gratefully acknowledged. It should go without saying that the views expressed in this volume are those of the authors and not necessarily those of the International Planned Parenthood Federation.

Chapter I

Latin American Family Planning in the 1970s

J. Mayone Stycos

International Population Program,
Cornell University

After a long, hungry childhood in the 1960s, Latin American family planning programs are, if not fat and sleek, at least being fed a minimum standard diet. Just recovering from the wonder of their own births, they are currently awed by the miracle of their growth and are looking to the future with the boundless optimism of adolescence. While psychologically salubrious, this outlook has led to a complacency about family planning programs that is unwarranted given the lack of clear evidence that national birth rates have been affected by organized family planning programs in the Western Hemisphere.° Moreover, since most family planning programs are low-key programs, designed to provide services for only a small minority of the population, and since most of the family planning financing comes from sources external to Latin America, the programs are generally both limited in impact and politically vulnerable.

The visitor to the typical clinic in a Latin American capital city will find it busy and crowded, with case loads often numbering in the thousands, indicating "a significant number of women" are receiving contraceptive services. In fact, in *national* terms the numbers are usually quite small, rarely exceeding 5 percent of the wo-

---

°There may be an exception in the case of Barbados. According to a recent analysis, "The spectacular decline in the birth rate in the 1960s was due mainly to the increasing use of contraceptives by the people of Barbados. It is the first country in the Western Hemisphere to receive government sanction and financial support for family planning." Moni Nag, "The Pattern of Mating Behaviour, Emigration and Contraceptives as Factors Affecting Human Fertility in Barbados," *Social and Economic Studies*, 20 (June 1971): 127.

men of reproductive age. Even more serious is the fact that this 5 percent represents a very special kind of minority. First of all, it is composed almost entirely of urban women, and urban women are more likely to limit their fertility with or without clinics. Many women who go to the clinics have already practiced contraception and are shopping for a better method or a reduction in cost; others would have eventually found the means to limit fertility in the absence of the clinics. Both types are more frequently found in the urban than in the rural areas. Thus, the "obviously sensible" strategy of locating the clinics at the places of the greatest demand—the cities—is to keep them away from the places of greatest need—the rural areas.

Closely related is the fact that most women attending clinics are over their peak period of fertility. Samples of the case loads of four Honduran clinics discussed in Chapter IV disclosed that the women had had an average of almost five pregnancies before going to the clinics; in the Dominican Republic (Chapter VI) over one-third of all new acceptors in the latter half of 1970 had five or more *living* children, and one-half had four or more; in Mexico City (Chapter II) women had an average 4.7 living children on first admission. While contraception will undoubtedly be of some individual assistance to such women, the impact on national birth rates will be much less than is commonly supposed.

On the whole then, not enough women are going to the clinics, and those who do go will not have the maximum impact on overall fertility rates. Essentially three reasons explain this situation. First, although Latin American women generally desire to have fewer children than they in fact have, their motivation for fertility reduction is not so intense that they can be expected to invest a high degree of personal effort in informing themselves, in seeking out services, or in diligently practicing contraception. This is probably true of significant proportions of urban women and of the majority of rural women. The evidence for these generalizations is contained in the considerable number of surveys conducted in Latin America during the 1960s, coupled with the few experimental studies designed to alter reproductive behavior. A good example is provided in Chapter V. In Bogota only 8 percent of a representative sample of women "likely to go to the clinic" in fact went even after personal visits from family planning educators who tried to persuade them to go to the clinics. That figure is only three percentage points higher than the control group which received no information or persuasion at all. This occurred in a city containing perhaps the best-attended birth control clinic in the world, a clinic that registered 1,000 new cases per month in 1970, in addition to 6,000 visits per month by old patients. These are, however, the women of the highest motivation and the highest past fertility. Most eligible women have considerably lower motivation.

It may be that large numbers of these eligible women can be effectively reached only after a poor nation achieves a higher level of economic and educational development. At the very least, however, medium-range programs of education on both population problems and family size problems could be carried out by the ministries of education, defense, and agriculture to reach deeper cognitive and motivational levels while the economy has a chance to develop. Instead, the "population problem" is almost invariably allocated to the ministry of health, which approaches the problem in the same fashion that it approaches an epidemic of the flu, except that it assigns family planning a lower priority.

A second reason for the minimal impact of family planning programs is the lack of commitment to these programs on the part of large sectors of the upper classes, often including the professional staffs of family planning programs. This stems partly from opposition to birth control programs from both the political right and left, an opposition that may water down the programs through ideological persuasion or political maneuvering. A good example in the public sector is the tendency to bury birth control programs in larger programs of maternal and child health where birth control efforts will not only be colorless but invisible. While it is doubtful that members of the far left and far right can be much influenced by public information programs, the moderates can be; and while the internationalization of family planning technical assistance cannot persuade the rightists and leftists, it can partially disarm them. Consequently, educating elites about national demographic problems is very much needed. None of this occurs in the public sector, and the private family planning efforts in this direction have tended to be sporadic and of miniscule proportions.

Finally, family planning programs are not strong enough because they are dominated by a basically conservative profession (the medical profession) utilizing a classical vehicle (the clinic) to supply services for people who are assumed to be sick and eager for a cure (the patients). This system would be bad enough if there were an adequate number of physicians, but hopelessly few are available to deal even with the serious problems of health facing poor countries. Whereas Mississippi has seventy-six physicians per 100,000 population, Central American countries average around twenty-five per

100,000. The supply of trained nurses is even more critical. The United States has two nurses for every physician, but most Latin American countries have two physicians for every nurse. Latin American physicians, moreover, are highly concentrated in urban areas. In Colombia, for example, less than one-third of the nation lives in the capital or in the provincial cities but over three-fourths of the physicians live there. In nations as diverse as Brazil, El Salvador, and Peru, while there are thirteen, seven, and nineteen physicians respectively for every 10,000 population in the cities, only one to two physicians exist per 10,000 outside of the cities. Thus, to tie family planning programs to doctors is to insist on urban services—again, putting the resources where the need is least.

There are growing signs too that many urban clinics are reaching saturation points, either because they are experiencing plateaus in demand or they have pushed the limits of their ability to supply, or both. In a number of countries, while the national totals of new acceptors are rising because new clinics continue to be opened in the provinces, the number of new acceptors in the older urban clinics is going into decline. Two of the reasons may be exhaustion of the supply of highly motivated women willing to go through the clinical routine in order to get a package of pills, as well as less motivation among the remaining "hard-core" women. As a clinic grows older, moreover, it grows more and more crowded with old patients on return visits—a fact that may give the clinic administrators the illusion of a prosperous program operating at top capacity while progressively discouraging new patients from attending. Thus, Venezuela sees four old patients for every new one and Brazil sees 5.5. In Chile, Colombia, and Mexico over three-fourths of the patients are old patients.

Even though the clinics are clogged with returning patients, many women who attend for the first time never attend for a second. In Keller's Mexico City study (Chapter II), for every 100 cases who enter, only 60 remain on the books at the end of a year. In Honduras, of the first 800 cases to enter government-sponsored Tegucigalpa clinics in 1970, Mundigo reports that 40 percent dropped out by the end of six months (Chapter IV).

At least four kinds of solutions to the limitations of clinical programs are indicated: first, internal clinic efficiencies to reduce waiting times and deploy medical skills more sparingly; second, stepped-up in-clinic educational efforts to reduce drop-out rates; third, more effective out-reach programs to bolster rates of new acceptors; and fourth, greater utilization of non-clinical channels of contraceptive supply.

Internal Clinic Efficiencies

Data subsequently discussed show that in both Mexico and Honduras there is a great deal of variation among clinics, not only with respect to numbers of new admissions but with respect to drop-out rates as well. These differences can be accounted for neither in terms of variation in contraceptives used nor the social or economic characteristics of the patients; rather, they seem clearly related to differences inherent in the personnel practices or procedure of the clinics. In Mexico reports of nervousness during the clinic experience varied by clinic from 24 to 54 percent, and complaints about treatment received varied from 2 percent to 17 percent. Detailed study of clinic procedure in Honduras disclosed how high motivation must be in order to attract and hold patients: a new patient waited an average of two and one-half hours before seeing a doctor for fifteen minutes. Even the patient going to a clinic for a fresh supply of pills waited two hours. While it could be argued that low income clientele expect little of public services anyway, the drop-out studies reported for Mexico and Honduras show that patients are by no means unaware of the inconveniences of the clinic. One-fourth of the Mexico City drop-outs gave "lack of time" as a reason for their not returning to the clinic and three-fourths of these implicated waiting time at the family planning center. Almost one in every ten complained of the way in which they were treated by the staff. The Honduran studies showed that in some instances, because of procedural inefficiencies, the doctors wait along with the patient. During a week of observation by a field worker in an urban Honduran clinic, one M.D. waited five hours for patients to be assigned to him. The typical physician, moreover, spends more time in form-filling than in examination and prescription. Many of the physician's routine tasks could be handled by a good auxiliary nurse. Certainly, on the average, physicians are not overworked. International Planned Parenthood Federation studies of family planning clinics in Brazil, Guatemala, Honduras, and Venezuela show that the number of new cases per hour of physician time in these countries is only 1.1, 1.4, 1.0, and 0.9 respectively. Clearly, the internal reorganization of clinic procedures is a fruitful area for both research and action.

In-clinic Education

Probably the greatest area of missed opportunity in family planning today refers to the chances for properly educating women who go to clinics. Any woman who is highly motivated enough to bring herself to the clinic and endure its routines is a woman who should subsequently serve as an educational agent for family planning among her peers. At the very least, she must remain a satisfied client, and what she learns will play a major role in determining her degree of satisfaction. Instead, as any observer of procedures in the average clinic can report, the typical educational effort, if it exists at all, is amateurish, formalistic, and often incomprehensible to its audience. Keller finds that only one-third to one-half of the patients followed up in five Mexico City clinics reported receiving information on side effects when they first visited the clinics; and fully one-half of the clinic drop-outs (as opposed to only one-fifth of those who remained active cases) later reported side effects. In Honduras only one-third of the drop-outs reported receiving an explanation of the methods and side effects, and of these only one-half said they understood the explanation. About one-half of all drop-outs had fears of the ill effects (largely cancer) of contraceptive practices, and one-third reported receiving negative information from friends that influenced their decision not to return to the clinic. In the urban community survey reported in Chapter III, no less than two-thirds of a representative sample of lower class women were afraid that contraceptives might be dangerous to their health.

Such data demonstrate the pressing need for more intensive and more imaginative approaches to educating the patient once she reaches the clinic. The assumption that she arrives ignorant should be replaced by the assumption that she arrives both misinformed and anxious about contraceptives.

Finally, inadequate as the educational effort is for the female, it is non-existent for the male, despite the fact that husband opposition is frequently mentioned as a reason for clinic defection. Special materials should be prepared for husbands (written materials, for example) that could be taken to him by the female patient. Again, this is an area ripe for action and evaluation.

Out-reach Programs

Imbued with a medical perspective that regards advertising as unethical, community education as irrelevant, and preventive medicine as uninteresting, medically directed family planning programs would not be expected to display much enthusiasm or ingenuity in the area of information and education. The government programs ignore this aspect altogether or rely on the traditional "health education" philosophy. This low-key, highly expensive approach depends heavily on the person-to-person approach so much a part of the doctor-patient medical mystique. It emphasizes social workers, "educators," and "promotors" who both talk woman-to-woman in the clinics and descend upon lower class communities in door-to-door canvasses. It plays down mass communications, community organizers, and grass-roots types of popular educators. Mass communications—radio, television, and printed media—offer great promise for educating Latin Americans. The studies reported in this volume concentrate on radio, which has the greatest potential of all because of its pervasiveness and economy. Three-fourths of the homes sampled in the Dominican Republic towns described in Chapter VI had radios, while in the low income Honduran sample two-thirds had radios, and most of the Honduran women listened more than three hours daily (Chapter III). Unlike exposure to television and newspapers, radio listening shows little variation by education, thus offering an excellent opportunity for democratizing information on family planning. Further, among the kind of highly transient, unneighborly low income urban populations described in Chapter III, radio may be a more effective diffusor of information than the fabled "grapevine," which can only work in communities with well-established networks of personal communication.

This is fine in theory, but does it work? Chapters III, V, and VI reporting on the evaluations of radio advertising in Honduras, Colombia, and the Dominican Republic demonstrate that it does. In all these countries the large majority of women heard the broadcasts, many of them learned about the location of a family planning clinic, and the case loads of the clinics increased significantly following the radio campaigns. In all countries, however, a differential response existed by type of city or clinic, suggesting that cultural and/or clinical variation also affects response. There is also some suggestion that younger women are especially responsive to this medium, an important matter for clinics that ordinarily attract higher parity women. It is also clear that all educational levels are reached, and, while not investigated, it can be assumed that men were reached as well as women. Further research is needed to determine to what extent differential programming (adapted to local conditions and to special target groups such as males, younger women, unmarried women, rural women, etc.) would produce even greater results.

Non-clinical Sources of Contraceptives
One solution to the many problems associated with clinical distribu-

tion of contraceptives is to bypass the clinics. The pharmacy has several advantages over the clinic as a supply source—anonymity, better service, no waiting, and no pelvic probing. It costs more, but the studies provide evidence that a significant minority of clinic drop-outs, despite their poverty, prefer to get contraceptives from the drug store. A program subsidizing commercial outlets for supplying materials at cost to poorer clients would probably be extremely popular in urban areas. Druggists could also receive special training in order better to refer problem cases to the clinics. In the rural areas, midwives could be utilized, in some instances trained to insert intra-uterine devices (IUD's) and refer problem cases. The armed forces, which conscript many rural men and often educate them, could include family planning education and services for them and for their wives. None of the studies contained in this volume addressed itself to these kinds of questions, but such questions should receive high priority for future research.

To move in the directions suggested as necessary to affect national birth rates will require the combined efforts of government and private programs. It will be the latter especially that should lead the way in the design and evaluation of new approaches, which, if successful, could eventually be adopted by governments. In this way the strides made in family planning in the 1970s might equal those made in the 1960s.

Chapter II

Patient Attrition in Five Mexico City Family Planning Clinics

Alan B. Keller

International Population Program,
Cornell University, and
Fundación para Estudios de la Población,
Mexico

As in many Latin American countries, Mexico's family planning clinics aim to help women avoid accidental pregnancies and to diminish the use of provoked abortion as a contraceptive method. Because relatively few Mexican women can financially afford medical advice or contraceptives from other reliable sources, these objectives are more likely to be achieved if patients who enroll at the clinics continue to return for supplies, medical checks, and advice. Many do not return. This study investigates the reasons why. It reports the results of research jointly undertaken in Mexico City in 1969 by the Fundación para Estudios de la Población (FEPAC) and the International Population Program, Cornell University.[1]

Among the relevant questions to which the inquiry was directed were:

1. What is the overall rate of desertion from Mexico City clinics?

2. How does desertion vary by contraceptive method, by clinic, by doctor, etc.?

3. What are the demographic and social-psychological correlates of desertion?

4. What reasons are given by patients for desertion?

5. What are the contraceptive histories of deserters following their defection from the clinic?

In an attempt to answer these questions a two-phase project was carried out. The first phase consisted of an analysis of clinic records containing attendance history, methods used, and demographic and medical data for each patient. The second phase involved a sample survey of clinic deserters and relatively long-term active patients. Before a discussion of the methodology and results of each of these phases, a brief consideration of the nature of the FEPAC program is appropriate.

The FEPAC System

The Fundación para Estudios de la Población is a private family planning organization founded in January 1966 and is affiliated with the International Planned Parenthood Federation.

At the end of 1969, FEPAC had thirty-six clinics with 43,428 registered patients, of which approximately 19,000 were registered in ten Mexico City clinics and 24,000 in twenty-six other clinics of the nation.

Each clinic is directed by a physician whose professional staff consists of social workers, nurses, and medical aides. There were a total of forty-seven doctors, fifty-seven social workers, twenty-five nurses, and twenty-seven receptionists employed in the thirty-six clinics and central offices. Each physician is responsible to the national executive director, who in turn is responsible to a board of directors.

The central offices of FEPAC are located in Mexico City and include, in addition to administrative personnel, a medical department that diagnoses the Papanicoulou tests (Pap smear), conducts medical education programs, and helps plan medical research; an education department that trains new staff and conducts educational programs for new patients and for professional and other public organizations; and a research and evaluation department.

The typical clinic is located in an apartment building or small house in an upper-lower class neighborhood.[2] It usually consists of a waiting room, a doctor's consulting room, a social worker's office, and occasionally an extra room utilized for meetings. All rooms are rather sparsely but pleasantly decorated with inexpensive local rugs, wall hangings, etc. The typical clinic carries between 1,000 and 2,000 patients on its registry.

Ideally, each new patient arriving at a clinic for the first time is given a registry number and shown films on family planning with a social worker in attendance to answer questions. The new patient then passes to the doctor who examines her, further explains the available contraceptive methods, advises against use of any that seem to be contraindicated in her case, and then leaves the patient to select a method.[3] Finally, the patient passes to a social worker who takes a demographic and socioeconomic history. Pap tests are done before insertion of IUD's and once every year thereafter. Pill and injection users are given Pap tests within one or two months after enrollment and annually thereafter. Injection users are expected to return to the clinic once every three months, pill users once a month, and IUD patients one month after insertion, three months later, six months later, and every six or twelve months thereafter, depending on the patient and the doctor.

Analysis of Clinic Records

The study was limited to the records of the five oldest and largest clinics of the Federal District (Mexico City). The records of every other patient enrolled in these clinics between November 1, 1966, and July 1, 1969, were coded for attendance history, methods used, and socio-demographic variables. Ten percent of the cases of each coder were recoded by a supervisor.

An examination of the clinic records of 300 women who had failed to continue treatment indicated that more than 90 percent of those who did not return within two months did not return within two years. Using this information the following definition was established: a patient is a clinic deserter if she is over two months late for her last appointment.

The resulting sample totaled 5,381 and, because many patients had entered after the July 1, 1969, cutoff date, consisted of one-third of all cases who had ever enrolled in the five clinics. Of the total sample, 3,175 were active patients and 2,206 were deserters; 39 percent of the total had accepted an oral contraceptive, 10 percent injections, and 51 percent the IUD.[4] Table II-1 shows that methods prescribed varied greatly by clinic.

Table II-1. Contraceptives Prescribed at Five Mexico City Clinics (in percent)

| Clinic | Contraceptive Prescribed | | | | Number of Cases |
	Oral	Injection	IUD	Total	
1	42	11	47	100	(2,112)
2	50	7	43	100	(1,212)
3	7	5	88	100	(753)
4	52	8	40	100	(727)
5	27	23	50	100	(567)

Socio-Demographic Profile

The large majority of patients at the five clinics are between 20 and 34 years of age. Comparison with 1960 census data for women 15 – 45 years of age in the Federal District shows that women in the youngest and oldest five-year age categories are underrepresented at the clinic (Table II-2).

Although the sample group is relatively young, the mean number of 4.7 living children is higher than the 4.14 reported by Benitez for a representative sample of fertile Mexico City women.[5] The Mexico City rates were the highest in a group of Latin American cities including Bogota; Buenos Aires; Caracas; Guatemala City; Panama City; Rio de Janeiro; San José, Costa Rica; and Santiago, Chile. As Table II-3 shows, almost one-half of the sample of clinic women had five or more children, and at every age had had more children than women in Benitez's sample. Nine percent of the patients ad-

---

Table II-2.   Age of Patients at Five Mexico City Clinics (in percent)

Age	Clinic Sample	1960 Census
15-19	3	22
20-24	23	20
25-29	30	17
30-34	24	15
35-39	15	13
40-44	5	13
Total	100	100

Table II-3.   Fertility of Clinic Patients and Fertile Federal District Females, by Age

Age	Living Children of Clinic Sample	Live Births of Federal District Women [a]
15-19	2.1	—
20-24	2.7	2.0
25-29	3.9	3.4
30-34	5.2	4.2
35-39	6.4	5.1
40-44	7.0	5.7

[a] Women with at least one live birth.

mitted to having one or more provoked abortions, though an even higher rate has been reported for Mexico in a study by Mateos Fournier.[6]

As Table II-4 shows, the educational levels of the clinic patients are virtually identical to Federal District women at the lower levels of primary school, but the clinic women bunch heavily at upper levels of elementary, with very few women having secondary schooling. Data on family income, though considerably less reliable than those on education, likewise indicate a distribution among clinic patients very similar to that found in the lower 70 percent of Federal District families.

Table II-4.   Education of Clinic Patients and Federal District Females (in percent)

Education	Clinic Sample	Federal District Women
None	12	13
1-3 years	26	23
4-6 years	56	39
7 years or more	6	25
Total	100	100

Data from a subsequent survey show that while 98 percent of the clinic patients are Roman Catholic only one-half go to church once a week, 25 percent go less than four times a year, and two-thirds state that they "almost never" take communion.[7]

Twenty-nine percent of the patients were born in areas of less than 50,000 inhabitants (about the same proportion as for Federal District residents in general), but most moved early in life to larger towns or directly to the Federal District.

Rates of Desertion

Abridged life tables were constructed to gauge rates of desertion from the five clinics. This technique yields a cumulative percentage of "survivors" at the end of various units of time based on what percentages the women who continue attending are of all women who have had the opportunity to attend at least as long as the given unit of time. The units of time chosen for the present study were: after one visit, and after three, six, nine, twelve, sixteen, twenty, twenty-four, thirty, and thirty-six months.[8]

Table II-5 presents the continuance rates of the total sample of 5,381 patients for each method group and for those patients who changed methods. For every 100 patients who enter the clinic, only 72 may be expected to remain active at the end of six months, 60 at the end of one year, 39 at the end of two years, and 21 at the end of three years. Thus desertion occurs most rapidly during the first six months, then diminishes during each major subsequent unit of time. This pattern has been reported in most clinical follow-up studies and may be a function of the early onset of side effects and other disagreeable aspects of clinic attendance method use; and it further may be a function of the consequent early reduction of the active patients to the most highly motivated group.

There are marked differences in rates of desertion by method.[9] IUD users remained for a longer time in the program, although in the long run differences between oral and IUD patients diminished. In other words, IUD and oral continuance rates do eventually even out, but this is due to an early and rapid drop off of oral patients followed by eventual stabilization and to a slow initial drop off of IUD patients followed by a more accelerated drop off. The result is a greater average number of months in treatment for IUD patients. Expected months of attendance for injection patients (whose small

Table II-5. Continuance Rates of Clinic Patients,
by Method (in percent)

Time	All Patients	IUD	Injection	Oral	Changers
After 1 visit	92	95	88	85	100
After 3 months	80	84	79	70	97
After 6 months	72	76	69	61	92
After 9 months	66	69	64	56	87
After 12 months	60	64	—	50	78
After 16 months	54	55	—	43	69
After 20 months	45	47	—	38	62
After 24 months	39	40	—	34	55
After 30 months	28	—	—	—	—
After 36 months	21	—	—	—	—
Number of cases	(5,381)	(2,543)	(321)	(1,939)	(578)

numbers unfortunately precluded analysis of patterns beyond the first nine months) fall between the other two.[10]

Continuance rates also vary according to clinic attended (Table II-6). That the lower rates in clinics 1 and 2 are not merely reflections of the differences in contraceptive methods employed in these clinics is indicated by the fact that there is less desertion in these clinics than would be expected according to use pattern. In all five clinics, desertion occurred soonest among oral users and latest among the IUD users. Clinic 4 had the highest rates of desertion for all three methods, while clinics 1 and 2 had the lowest rates in all methods.

Surprisingly, clinics 1 and 2 had the highest patient/doctor ratios of the five clinics, and clinic 1 was especially overcrowded. The high levels of desertion in clinic 4 may be related to the facts that the clinic was on a part-time schedule, the doctor was prone to arrive late for work, and the facility was crowded. The hypothesis that women might desert because of uneasiness about being examined by male doctors was not supported, since the doctors in the two clinics with least desertions were males and those in the three with most desertions were females.

Table II-6. Actual (A) and Expected (E) Continuance Rates of Clinic Patients, by Clinic (in percent)

Time	Clinic 1		2		3		4		5	
	A	E	A	E	A	E	A	E	A	E
After 1 visit	93	91	94	90	87	94	87	89	92	90
After 3 months	84	78	83	77	76	83	72	76	75	77
After 6 months	76	69	76	69	70	75	62	67	65	68
After 9 months	71	64	71	63	64	68	56	62	55	63
After 12 months	65	58	65	57	59	63	49	56	50	57
After 16 months	57	50	58	49	50	54	39	48	36	49
After 20 months	51	43	51	43	42	46	35	41	—	—
After 24 months	45	38	45	37	34	39	30	36	—	—
Number of cases	(2,122)		(1,212)		(753)		(727)		(567)	

NOTE: The expected continuance rates by clinic were derived by taking the observed continuance rates for each method and projecting these rates for each clinic, according to the distribution of methods used in these clinics.

In sum, desertion rates are high and vary markedly by contraceptive method and clinic, but neither method nor other general characteristics such as patient/doctor ratio account for clinic variation.

Demographic Variables and Desertion

The demographic characteristics of deserters and active patients were compared, and, since some deserters had attended longer than some of the active cases, deserters within three months and deserters within one year were compared to active patients with at least two years of attendance. Neither age nor number of children is related to desertion. Consequently, within the range of patients served by the FEPAC program, clinic and method factors rather than demographic characteristics of the patients seem to be related to desertion (Table II-7).

Follow-up Interviews with Patients and Deserters

To investigate the causes, results, and consequences of desertion, a one-hour interview was developed that included questions on socioeconomic and demographic characteristics, on reasons for not returning to the clinic, and on contraceptive and pregnancy histories following desertion.[11] The interviewers were twenty female advanced social work students who had excelled in classroom and fieldwork performance. This group received a ten-day training program that included lectures on population problems; the FEPAC program; psychological, moral, sociological, and medical aspects of family planning; the contents of the interviews; and techniques of interviewing. Demonstrations of good and bad interviewing techniques were given, practice interviews were conducted by each interviewer in front of the group, and each interviewer was sent to the field to conduct two acceptable interviews before she could join the interview team.

The initial goal of the research team was to interview 1,000 deserters and 100 active patients with at least twelve months of attendance. Because it was anticipated that many women would not be located, the names and addresses of 1,848 deserters and 222 active patients were randomly drawn from the 5,381 cases coded in the clinics.

Eight percent of the deserters and 3 percent of the actives were

Table II-7. Number of Living Children and Age, by Desertion
Status (in percent)

Number of Living Children	Active Patients	Deserters
1-3	33	38
4-5	31	30
6-7	20	18
8 or more	16	14
Total	100	100
Age		
Under 25	23	28
25-29	28	28
30-34	25	23
35-39	17	15
40 and over	7	6
Total	100	100

discarded because they lived more than fifteen miles from Mexico City. Another 18 percent of the deserters and 23 percent of the attenders were eliminated because they lived far away from other potential interviewees (but *not* farther from the clinics than many, if not most, of those ultimately interviewed).

Twenty-three percent of the remaining deserters and 19 percent of the actives were found to have given the clinic false addresses. An additional 19 percent of the former and 12 percent of the latter group had moved and new addresses could not be obtained. Refusals were encountered in less than 3 percent of the deserters and 2 percent of the actives. The sample of women interviewed represents 53 percent of the deserters and 67 percent of the active patients whom the interviewers actually tried to contact.[12]

Because of these problems in locating cases, the work was terminated after interviews were conducted with 703 deserters and 110 active patients. Seventy-six percent of the active patient interviewees had attended the clinics between one and two years, and 24 percent had attended more than two years. Among deserters, 79 percent deserted within the first year, 16 percent during the second, and 5 percent after the second.[13]

The number of interviewees from each clinic roughly approximates the relative sizes of the clinic populations, and the methods used by the interviewees tend to mirror the use patterns by clinic. The socioeconomic and demographic characteristics of the interviewees closely resemble those reported for the universe of 5,381.

Contraception after Desertion

Interest in the consequences of desertion prompted an attempt to classify contraceptive use after desertion. Several definitions were utilized. Effective methods (sterilization, IUD, oral, injection) were those reported in the *Journal of the Mexican Society of Obstetrics and Gynecology* as having a failure rate of less than 20 percent per year in Mexico.[14] Regular use meant constant use after leaving the clinic except to achieve a desired pregnancy or recuperation from illness.

By these definitions, 41 percent of the deserters continued with regular use of effective methods; 42 percent used no methods; and 17 percent were characterized by occasional use of ineffective methods, irregular use of effective methods, or regular use of ineffective methods (the great majority in the first category). Optimistically stated, 58 percent of the deserters are still to some extent protected by contraception, but pessimistically stated 59 percent run a rather high risk of becoming pregnant.

When deserters were divided between those who had deserted one year or less prior to the interview and those who had deserted more than one year prior, virtually no difference was found in the quality of contraception practiced. If a deserter continued at all with effective contraception, she was inclined to do so for at least two years. Conversely, if the deserter did not continue with effective contraception in the first year after desertion, she was unlikely to begin again in the second. Finally, deserters who did not utilize effective methods after desertion tended to have had fewer children than women who did (40 percent of the women who did not use effective methods had three or fewer children, as compared with 29 percent of the women who did use effective methods). Hence, although desertion itself proved unrelated to the number of living children, contraceptive behavior after desertion showed a rather strong relationship to fertility with women of lower fertility less inclined to contracept possibly because of desires to have more children or less desire to avoid having more. Equally important, however, is the fact that the majority of non-users of effective methods after desertion had more than three children.

Rather pronounced differences in contraceptive usage are seen by method.[15] As Table II-8 indicates, IUD patients in all five clinics were much more likely than users of either oral or injectable contraceptives to continue regular use of a reliable method after desertion. Any variation between clinics was found to be a function of differences in proportions of users of contraceptive method. The differences by method grow when deserters are divided by time of desertion. The percentages of IUD deserters who used effective contraceptives are identical for women who defected recently and women who defected more than a year ago. Among oral patients, however, 25 percent fewer women continued use in the second year of desertion than in the first. The persistence of IUD users in effective contraceptive efforts is, as might be expected, a function of their retaining the IUD's received in the clinic (Table II-9).[16]

The majority of the 119 deserters using a method requiring supplies (pills, injections, cream, condoms, etc.) received them directly from a non-medical source without medical attention (Table II-10).[17]

While 80 percent of the women said the new source of supply was closer to their residence and 87 stated that they needed less time to get to the new source, 73 percent admitted that supplies were more expensive from the new source. When asked why they

---

Table II-8.   Contraceptive Use after Desertion by Previous Contraceptive Experience (in percent)

	Regular Use, Effective Method	Partial Protection	No Use of Any Method	Total	Number of cases
IUD	62	12	26	100	(321)
Oral	22	23	55	100	(342)
Injection	29	21	50	100	(28)

Table II-9.   Contraceptive Use after Desertion for Women Who Continue to Contracept

	Percent Using Same Method	Number of Continuing Contraceptors
IUD	78	(238)
Oral	42	(154)
Injection	14	(14)

Table II-10.   Source of Supplies among Contracepting Deserters
Requiring Supplies (in percent)

Source	
Pharmacy	61
Private doctor	19
Doctor in hospital	8
Doctor in clinic (not FEPAC)	2
Friends	4
Other	6
Total	100
Number of cases	(119)

Table II-11.   Reasons for Preferring Source Outside Clinic,
for Clinic Deserters (in percent)

Reason	
Less time in waiting	34
Rumors about the clinic	31
Cheaper	11
Bad attention in the clinic	10
Less time in transportation	9
Other	5
Total	100

went to the new source, the women gave the responses listed in
Table II-11.

Pregnancy and Desertion

During the period of clinic attendance, 4 percent of the future deserters became pregnant compared to 3 percent of the active patients. In neither group were the expected yearly failure rates of the
methods employed greatly exceeded. After desertion, however,
fully one-third of the deserters had become pregnant by the time of
the interview. The rate for actives remained at 3 percent. Those
who had post-desertion pregnancies were generally relatively high
parity women. Of 240 deserters who became pregnant, only 31 stat-

ed that they left the clinic in order to get pregnant, but 77 said that the post-desertion pregnancy was intentional—statements that may be *ex post facto* attempts to rationalize what actually occurred.

Patients' Explanations of Desertion

During the interviews deserters were first asked "Why did you not return to the clinic?" and then thoroughly probed in order to elicit possible multiple reasons as well as the chronological ordering of those reasons. Several types of answers were encountered: single reasons ("I wanted to get pregnant."); chronological chains of reasons ("First I had to leave town. Then when I got back, I got pregnant."); and non-chronological, multiple reasons ("I had to wait too long, and the receptionist was rude to me."). Only first and second reasons were coded.

Before the study began, several of the clinic doctors predicted that deserters would prove to be those who purposely left the program to get pregnant, on the one hand, and those who were no longer exposed to conception on the other. Although this conclusion may be true of the few deserters who return to the clinics for IUD extractions, only 4 percent of all deserters gave the desire to become pregnant as a reason for leaving the clinic, and only 6 percent mentioned sterility or low risk of pregnancy (Table II-12).

Pressure of time was the most frequently mentioned reason. This category included statements that the respondent had too much to do at home to permit her going to the clinic (100 respondents), that she had to work (45), that she had to wait too long in the clinic (19), or that she had to spend too much time in transportation (13). Since the declaration of those women who said that they have too much to do in the home generally implicates waiting time in the clinic ("With all I have to do here I can't be spending time there."), and since 19 of the 45 women who cited having to work also indicates that waiting times may be a factor in not returning ("I have to work, and my free hours don't give me enough time to attend."), waiting time in the clinic was directly or indirectly suggested as a reason for desertion by over three-fourths of the 177 women citing time pressures. The remaining one-fourth stated that transportation took too much time or that the coincidence of their employment and clinic schedules precluded clinic attendance.

Side effects were almost exclusively mentioned as a first reason, and often other reasons followed. A very common experience was simply based on side effects ("I had headaches and I was gaining

Table II-12.   First and Second Reasons for Deserting Clinic

Reason	Number	Percent
Pressures of time	177	26
Side effects	165	24
Accidental pregnancy	150	22
Left city	73	11
Laziness, lack of will	69	10
Unable to receive treatment, maltreatment by staff	58	8
Objections of others	56	8
Lack of money	44	6
Recuperation from illness or accident	43	6
Separation from or death of spouse, sterile	38	6
Belief in bad effects of contraception	35	5
Desired pregnancy	34	4
Went to another source	28	4
Fear of censure	16	2
Other reasons	88	13
Number of women giving a reason	(680)	

weight. I began to believe that the methods were dangerous and I didn't go back."); but in others the deserter experienced the side effect in combination with other negative experiences ("I felt very nervous and went back to the clinic. They told me it was natural but that didn't make me feel better.").

Most replies concerning accidental pregnancies came as second reasons, demonstrating (as do the data on sequences of reasons) that the pregnancy typically *resulted from* desertion for some other reason ("I kept having headaches and after I quit going to the clinic I got pregnant.").

Since interviewees were in Mexico City and at the time of the interview still had not returned to the clinic, leaving the city was seldom the most recent reason given for desertion. Rather this occurrence was generally given as the first reason of a series. The frequency of this reason signals the high incidence in the groups served by the clinics of prolonged visits to outlying areas and the threat such a pattern poses to continuing clinic attendance.

Maltreatment by staff usually referred to a situation in which a patient was shamed by being lectured in front of other patients for arriving late for appointments. Such women were reluctant to return for fear of once again undergoing this type of experience. Interviewees who complained of being unable to receive attention generally had arrived late for an appointment or had not arrived during their menstrual periods and felt that they were denied an adequate explanation of why they could not receive treatment.

Opposition of others (generally the spouse) was a first reason in about one-half the cases who mention this situation and a second reason in the other half. In the latter group, the opposition was not forcefully expressed until the patient had an unfortunate experience with the method or the clinic ("I had irregular bleeding, and when my husband found out he wouldn't let me go back anymore."). Consequently the incidence of strong opposition of others *before* use actually began was approximately one-half of the 8 percent who listed opposition of others as a reason. The opposition that developed after clinic attendance generally was due to suspicion of the methods after bad personal experiences ("After I started getting the headaches, he decided that what he had heard was true and he didn't want me to go back."). Except for the fact that this opposition was attributed to others, these cases could have been included in the category "belief in bad effects of contraceptives or loss of faith in clinic."

Some of the reasons offered—self-diagnosed laziness or lack of will—explicitly suggest a motivational problem; others imply it, at least in the sense that highly motivated women might be expected to surmount such problems as time pressures, side effects, problems in the clinic, or objections of others. However, the clinics also appear to be contributing heavily to desertion through such factors as waiting time, financial policy (not all women knew that the service can be free), and failure to educate patients adequately.

The few differences in reasons by method are shown in Table II-13. Users of the IUD were most inclined to cite the time factor as their reason for not returning—a probable indication of their having to wait longer because of the need to be seen by the doctor at each visit. In addition, IUD patients were more inclined to cite laziness or lack of will. This may be due to an inclination on the part of many IUD patients, partly because of their belief that they are protected against pregnancy, to avoid the unpleasantness or inconvenience of waiting in the clinic. Being more assured, they are less tolerant. Several openly declared, "Maybe I'll go back if I have any trouble, but if not, why should I bother?" For users of the injection and pill, however, the most frequently offered reason was a desire to escape side effects of the method itself.[19] However, many of their number also were driven by the time factor to other sources or to giving up protection altogether.

* **Table II-13.   Reasons for Desertion, by Method (in percent)**

Reason	Method		
	IUD	Injection	Oral
Left city	13	11	8
Pressures of time	33	22	20
Side effects	14	29	32
Laziness, lack of will	18	13	3

An examination of reasons for desertion by clinic revealed few differences, and several of those found were largely accounted for by variations in methods prescribed by the different clinics.

Finally, when reasons were examined in relation to time of desertion, only two differences were observed. Side effects were listed as a reason for desertion during the first year of attendance more frequently than in the second or third year, and more frequently in the first few than the later months of the first year—a finding in accord with medical observations about the typical times of onset of most side effects from contraceptive use. On the other hand, desire for a pregnancy was more commonly offered as a reason for desertion after a year at the clinic—attesting to the attendance of women when purpose is primarily to space rather than to terminate pregnancies.

Other Influences on Desertion

Since many factors bearing on the decision not to return to the clinic might not be consciously recognized because they are repressed or not recalled, a series of direct questions on desertion was included in the interview. These were also asked of the sample of respondents who still attend the clinics. However, the nature of the active patients sample limited the possibility of differences between the groups. Although the active patients had attended the clinic for at least a year, some had not attended as long as some deserters. A comparison between attenders of three or more years, for example, and deserters who leave before eighteen months would have been preferable. Nevertheless, since the active patients had a higher average number of months of attendance than the deserters and since the majority of them had attended longer than the majority of deserters, some differences were expected, but few were found. Table II-14 presents the variables that showed some relationship to desertion. Inconsistent with the expectation that female employment encourages contraceptive usage was the finding that women who worked were somewhat more likely than nonworking women to desert. Since the working women were no more prone than other deserters to utilize contraception after desertion, they were also probably less effective contraceptors than nonworking women. Since the respondents were not asked about current work status, the conclusion cannot be made with assurance that employment leads to time pressures that make waiting in the clinic difficult. It will be remembered, however, that forty-five deserters gave exactly that reason for their desertion.

Table II-14. Variables Related to Desertion

	Active Patients	Deserters
Percent who had ever worked outside home for one year or more	59	69
Percent who had received service for births and other medical attention	46	38
Percent who had previously used a clinic-recommended contraceptive method	24	17
Percent with someone to take care of children during clinic visits	54	45
Number of cases	(680)	(107)

The larger percentage of active patients who had received maternal care services might suggest that continuing clinic attendance is related to familiarity with clinic atmosphere and medical procedure. Similarly, familiarity with effective contraceptives showed a relationship to continuing attendance. Deserters were less likely than attenders to have someone with whom they could leave their children during clinic visits.

The area of communication between spouses, found to be important for effective contraception in Puerto Rico (Hill, Stycos, Back),[20] appears also to be related to desertion in Mexico. A higher percentage of active Mexican patients than deserters claimed to have discussed with their spouses both whether or not the spouse wanted more children and future use of contraception. Moreover, a higher percentage of deserters than active patients claimed not to have discussed either topic.

While reported agreement of the husband with clinic attendance and/or method use was typical among both active patients and deserters, about one-fourth of each group felt that their husbands would oppose such action.

No differences were found between active patients and deserters on the opinions of other relatives about contraception and clinic attendance. Friends of the members of both groups generally were in favor of clinic attendance and contraceptive use, but sizeable minorities in each group did not discuss such matters with their friends.

Finally, an effort was made to assess overall levels of social support encountered by the respondents. At one end of the continuum was the patient whose husband, friends, and relatives were completely in favor of her contraceptive efforts, and at the other end the woman whose efforts were unknown or opposed by all these individuals. Somewhat more of the active patients than deserters fell into the former category, and relatively few individuals in either group fell into the latter. Fully 80 percent of the members of both groups lived in environments of mixed or total support.

Table II-15 demonstrates no differences between active patients and deserters in ideal family size or desire for more children. Very few wanted more children, and the mean ideal family size for the two groups was 3.75 children. This is somewhat lower than the 4.1 average reported for Mexico City by Stycos,[21] suggesting that women who had actually reached the clinic were motivated toward relatively small families.

Nevertheless, since one-third of those who did not want more children declared that they would be happy or indifferent if they were to have another child, close to one-half of both active patients and deserters manifested some degree of motivation in favor of enlarging families that already averaged 4.7 children.

Clinic Experiences

Table II-16 relates desertion to six aspects of clinic attendance. The factor bearing the strongest relationship is the patient's feeling nervous in the clinic. Unfortunately no probes were included to discover exactly what this complaint implied, although analysis by clinic (see below) does give some clues. Waiting time shows a slight relation to desertion, and in both groups long waiting times were reported. Coupled with the earlier datum that long waiting times were frequently offered as a reason for desertion, a crucial factor in the explanation of desertion may involve the clinic itself.

Complaints about costs or treatment by staff do not appear strongly related to desertion. However, since 8 percent of all deserters cited some form of maltreatment by staff, and 6 percent cited lack of money as reasons for desertion, the importance of complaints shown in Table II-16 should not be dismissed.

A strong association exists between desertion and reported side effects. One-fifth of the active patients but just under one-half of the deserters reported side effects. It should be recalled that one-fourth of all deserters listed side effects as a cause of their not returning to

Table II-15. Family Size Preference, by Desertion Status (in percent)

Motivating Factor	Active Patients	Deserters
Ideal number of children		
1-3	41	43
4	38	38
5	11	11
6 or more	10	8
Total	100	100
Wife wants more children	14	19
Husband wants more children	53	

Table II-16. Factors Affecting Dissatisfaction with Clinic, by Desertion Status (in percent)

	Active Patients	Deserters
Felt nervous in clinic	28	41
Waited 90 minutes or more in clinic	64	72
Lived 20 or more blocks from clinic	54	59
Traveled 30 minutes or more to clinic	46	48
Complained about treatment by staff	6	10
Complained about clinic fees	4	5

the clinic. In view of the importance of side effects, Table II-17 concerning side effects by method and Table II-18 concerning education on this and other matters given in the clinic are most revealing. Women who reported not having received advice from the clinic

Table II-17.   Reported Side Effects among Deserters, by Method
(in absolute numbers)

Reported Side Effect	Method	
	IUD	Oral
Hemorrhage	46	16
Menstrual irregularity	23	3
Headaches	11	79
Gain in weight	3	15
Swellings, blotches, or inflammations	5	15
Nausea	7	33
Vaginal discharge	8	0
Pain in uterus	18	1
Ulcer in reproductive tract	4	2
Nervousness	12	58
Number of users	(361)	(399)
Number of users reporting one or more side effects	(130)	(172)

Table II-18.   Clinic Education and Susceptibility to Rumor,
by Desertion Status (in percent)

	Active Patients	Deserters
Received information from clinic about side effects:		
Among those who had side effects	75	50
Among those who had no side effects	44	29
Received information from clinic that other methods were available	93	76
Heard rumors about possible side effects	42	53
Among those heard rumors, percent who believed them	22	43

about side effects were more likely to desert than those who had—especially if they actually experienced side effects.[22] Further-more, rather strong differences between active patients and desert-ers were noted concerning whether information on the availability of other methods in the clinic was received. While a relationship ob-tains between desertion and lack of this information, the absolute numbers of women stating that they were told about other meth-ods are much higher in both groups than the numbers acknowledg-ing receipt of information about side effects. Thus, the clinics ap-pear more successful in conveying the former than the latter mes-sage.

An important by-product of education in the clinic should be to build resistance against negative rumors concerning the clinic and contraception. As expected, deserters were more likely to have heard, and especially to have believed, such rumors. Table II-19 shows that the majority of rumors concerned the health dangers of practicing contraception. Conspicuously absent were rumors depict-ing the clinic in political terms. Three-fourths of those who heard ru-mors cite family members as the source, 38 percent mention non-family members, and 13 percent mention a priest. That only 5 percent mention the mass media may be due to question wording that oriented responses toward individuals.

Knowledge of the existence, effectiveness, and degree of safety to health of at least two effective methods was viewed as particularly important for continued clinic attendance since a woman who en-counters problems with the prescribed method needs to know an-

Table II-19.   Rumors concerning Clinics and Methods

	Number of Citations
Clinic or contraceptives harm health of women	228
Clinic violates laws of Roman Catholic Church	113
Clinic supplies pills that harm health	58
Clinic harms health of future generations	27
Clinic supplies IUD, which harms health	17
Clinic gives injections, which harm health	7
Clinic disobeys laws of Mexico	2

NOTE: Several questions yielded information about rumors: "What have you heard about these clinics?" "What have you heard about these methods?" "What do your husband, friends, and relatives think about the methods?"

other adequate one is available. Forty-one percent of the total sample had such information, but 86 percent had accurate knowledge of one effective method.[23] The importance of knowing two or more effective methods is borne out in the relationship between continuing attendance and knowledge of two or more effective methods (Table II-20).

Table II-20. **Knowledge of Methods, by Desertion Status (in percent)**

	Active Patients	Deserters
Knowledge of two or more effective methods	56	38
Attribute knowledge of two or more effective methods to clinic	35	18
Attribute knowledge of no effective method to clinic	10	31

Further, fully 71 percent of the respondents attribute knowledge of an effective method to the clinic. Thus a higher percentage of the interviewees have learned about an *effective* method in the clinic than the percentage of the population at large knows of any method.[24] A relationship also obtains between attribution of knowledge to the clinic and continuing attendance.

Clinic Variations

Neither the facts known about the clinics before the study began (such as the doctor/patient ratio) nor conscious reasons for desertion adequately explain the variance in desertion by clinic. Consequently replies to the direct questions about service were studied by clinic.

As Table II-21 suggests, clear differences between clinics were found among the proportions of women who felt nervous in the clinic situation.[25] To a certain extent, the high incidence in clinic 3 may be explained by the fact that this clinic had the highest proportion of IUD patients. It may be that IUD patients, who are required to undergo a physical examination at each visit, are more nervous in the clinic situation. However, method use does not fully account for the inter-clinic variance.

Reported waiting times also varied by clinic. While the clinic with the highest patient/doctor ratio and the largest number of registered patients had the second highest incidence of reported waits of ninety minutes or more, the clinic with the lowest incidence had the second highest patient/doctor ratio. The clinic with the highest incidence of lengthy waiting was operating only half time. Finally, differences in reported waiting times bore no relationship to the proportions of interviewees using each method.

Table II-21. **Factor Affecting Dissatisfaction with Clinic, by Clinic (in percent)**

	Clinic				
	1	2	3	4	5
Felt nervous in the clinic	37	24	54	44	34
Waited 90 minutes or more	78	35	74	83	73
Lived 30 or more blocks from clinic	81	37	43	51	57
Complained about treatment by staff	17	2	3	7	13
Complained about fees	4	2	4	7	11

NOTE: Percentages are of all interviewees from each clinic.

Although distance from clinic and time in transportation proved to have little relationship to desertion,[26] most women who stated that they deserted for this reason were from clinic 1, where the highest percentage of patients live more than thirty blocks away from the clinic.

This clinic also registered the highest percentage of complaints over treatment by staff, possibly because it has the highest patient/doctor ratio. On the other hand, clinic 2, with only one doctor and the second largest patient load in the FEPAC system, registered a very low number of complaints.

Data on specific personnel mentioned in complaints suggest an extraordinary situation in clinic 1 involving all personnel, but especially the receptionists. Indeed, in general, the role of the receptionist appears very important. Of seventy-seven specific complaints, close to one-half (thirty-two) concerned the receptionist; fifteen the doctor; fourteen the social worker; sixteen the nurse. Complaints over fees also varied by clinic and show little relation to other types of complaints.

Differences by clinic in the incidence of reported side effects are

Table II-22.   Information, by Clinic (in percent)

	Clinic				
	1	2	3	4	5
Received information about side effects	35	45	50	42	41
Received information that other methods were available at clinic	76	77	79	78	85
Believed rumor, among those who had heard it	41	34	36	45	33
Cited clinic as source of information for two or more effective methods known	19	24	13	37	21
Cited clinic as source of information for no methods known	33	25	23	27	30

NOTE: Percentages are of all interviewees from each clinic.

also apparent, but the differences are not great. One other interesting possibility emerges: clinic 1 also had about the poorest record of the five in transmitting information to its patients (Table II-22). Other clinics had less consistent patterns. Equally impressive, however, is the low level of success that all clinics had in communicating.

As may be observed, this review of clinic performance factors, while adding to the overall picture of the causes of clinic differences in desertion, does not afford an entirely consistent model of the causes of such differences. Clinic 1, for example, with the highest patient/doctor ratio and one of the poorer overall records on the performance variables, nevertheless had, along with clinic 2, the lowest desertion rate. Factors unmeasured in the present study probably influence desertion levels by clinic in conjunction with some or all of the measured ones.

Summary

Two characteristics of Mexico's FEPAC patients should be re-emphasized—one characteristic is a favorable indicator of the program's potential role in reducing the rate of population growth; the other characteristic is a somewhat unfavorable indicator. The first is that the clinics do not serve only women who were already effective contraceptors before attending the clinics. Only 20 percent of the sample had had any previous experience with effective contraceptive methods. The second is that although demographically the patients are quite representative of lower income Mexico City women in the appropriate age range, one important group is underrepresented in the clinic population—low parity women of any age. In spite of the fact that promotion of clinic services is given mated women without regard to parity, it is disproportionately those with already large families who enroll in the program. Since the women studied are from Mexico's largest, most industrialized, and least traditionalist city, there is no reason to expect the pattern to differ in provincial city and rural clinics.

For the FEPAC clinics as a whole, about three-quarters of the patients remained active at the end of six months, 60 percent by the end of a year, 39 percent at the end of two years, one-fifth at the end of three years. Thus most desertion occurred initially and diminishes rapidly over time.

Desertion in the early months was more frequent among pill than IUD patients, with injection patients falling between. In the second year, however, IUD desertion rates are somewhat higher than pill rates, and the survivorship levels become more similar. The result of the initially lower desertion rates of IUD patients was, nevertheless, a higher average of months of attendance by IUD patients—a difference observed in studies in the United States and Taiwan. Desertion was also found to vary by clinic in a manner not explainable by differences in method use; nor was it found to have a strong relation to any of the demographic variables examined.

Analysis of contraceptive practice after desertion confirmed that clinic desertion was not tantamount to method desertion, since 58 percent may be considered as continuing some contraceptive activity after desertion. Sixty-four percent of IUD patients but only 22 percent of pill patients were well protected after desertion, largely because most of the IUD patients continued use of the IUD after leaving the clinic. Over one-third of all deserters but 60 percent of the unprotected became pregnant during the first year of desertion. Lower rates of desertion among IUD patients may be related to the lower reported incidence of side effects with the IUD, fewer rumors in circulation about the IUD, and the need for fewer visits to the clinic by IUD users.

The particular clinic the patients attend also bears a strong relationship to desertion. However, neither directly observable characteristics of the clinics, such as patient/doctor ratio, nor indices of clinic performance, such as waiting time and success at educating patients, afford a consistent explanation of clinic variation. Perhaps other factors (unmeasured in the present study) such as ability and/or sex of the doctors are involved.

Since only about 6 percent of all deserters were either sterile or unexposed to conception, 5 percent deserted to become pregnant, and 4 percent were still recuperating from an illness or injury, only about 15 percent can be said to have deserted for reasons beyond the control of the clinics.

Ambivalence about having more children was characteristic even among rather high parity and relatively highly motivated women. At least 45 percent of the women sampled want more children. It is plausible to assume that in many of these women motivation is sufficiently low to permit almost any untoward experience or simple lack of firm moral support from others to lead to desertion. Thus, desertion may be both a function of low motivation and unpleasant clinic or method experience. Fully one-quarter of the deserters directly or indirectly gave clinic "waiting time" as their reason for desertion. The fact that working women are more likely to desert and that high percentages of active patients also say they have to wait long periods suggests that this reason is not a mere rationalization employed by the deserters. Fourteen percent claimed they failed to return to the clinic because of maltreatment by the staff or the inability to pay fees.

Another important factor bearing on desertion is inadequate or inaccurate information about contraceptives and thus about possible side effects.

Lack of communication between spouses bears a rather strong relationship to desertion, and opposition of the spouse may be present in from 20 to 25 percent of the couples served by the clinics.

Accidental pregnancy proved to be an almost insignificant *reason* for desertion. It seems plausible that other studies citing accidental pregnancy as an important reason for desertion when the population studied was using reliable contraceptive methods are based on deficient interviewing techniques.

Chapter III

Health and Family Planning in a Honduran Barrio

J. Mayone Stycos
Parker G. Marden

International Population Program,
Cornell University

In the summer of 1968 a team from the Cornell University International Population Program carried out an action-research project in four low income barrios in Tegucigalpa, Honduras.[1] The project was designed to develop baseline information on knowledge, attitudes, and decision-making processes concerning health and family planning; and to assess the manner and extent to which an educational campaign using the mass media could influence the demand for family planning services among an urban, low income group.

The research was conducted in four contiguous barrios—Las Crucitas, Los Profesores, Colonia Obrera, and El Pastel—in the northwest part of Comayaguela, which forms the capital district of Honduras together with its larger twin city of Tegucigalpa. (For simplicity, the entire study area will hereafter be identified as "Las Crucitas" after the largest of the four barrios and the health center contained within it.) The decision to study these four barrios was based on several criteria. First, the four barrios form an identifiable ecological area with a population of sufficient size to test the study's hypotheses adequately. Second, the area contains a major governmental health center that provides a range of health services, including family planning. While Las Crucitas Health Center served a much larger geographic area, it seemed reasonable to test various research hypotheses among a population to which its services were conveniently available. Third, all preliminary indicators, available from a variety of sources including the Health Center, identified the study population as one characterized by high fertility, low socioeconomic status, and high migration. These features are typical of much of Tegucigalpa-Comayaguela's population and are relevant to the research.

The initial project involved a complete enumeration of the population living in the four barrios. Working from maps of the thirty-five-block area provided by the City Planning Department, this enumeration identified 1,717 households, estimated the population as 10,300, and provided other basic demographic and socioeconomic data. (The size of the population exceeded the highest estimates based upon earlier studies conducted within the four barrios.)

The enumeration also provided a frame from which four 25 percent samples of households could be drawn. One of the samples (A) was used to gather basic information about the population of Las Crucitas, and two samples (B and C) were reserved to test hypotheses on the use of mass media in disseminating health and family planning information. A fourth sample (D) was not used. Within each of the thirty-five blocks in the study area, all households were randomly assigned to one of the four samples.

Following the enumeration, a thirty-minute, census-type questionnaire was administered to the 422 households assigned to Sample A. (For convenience, this study is referred to as the "census" here.) It collected basic information on each member of the household (closely following the format and procedures of the 1961 Honduran census), elicited a migration history of the head of the household, and investigated attitudes toward health services. Completed census interviews were obtained from 400, or 95 percent, of the households drawn for the sample. Samples B and C each consisted of 425 households.

While the interviews in Sample B were being conducted, two subsamples of the households in Sample A, the "census" sample, were chosen for more intensive reinterviewing. One subsample was used for a study of fertility and family structure (A_1), and the other was used for a study of fertility, family income, and decision making (A_2). Since both studies contained many identical questions about fertility and family planning, much of the information presented here is based on the combined subsamples. The families selected in the two subsamples met three criteria: 1) the male partner was present, 2) the wife was within the reproductive ages 15—44 years, and 3) she had at least one child.

In addition to these surveys, an analysis of attendance rates at the family planning clinics at San Felipe Hospital and Las Crucitas Health Center was undertaken; the Las Crucitas Health Center was observed for a four-week period; and a community study of the barrios was carried out by a Cornell graduate student participant observer.

Las Crucitas and Its Population

Physical Environment

The four barrios (hereafter referred to simply as "the barrio") that compose the study area identified as Las Crucitas form an ecological area bounded by steep hills, a large cemetery, a stream, and the main highway between Tegucigalpa and San Pedro Sula. The area spreads across several hills located just above the capital district's main market area, where many of the area's residents work.

Table III-1 shows that less than one-third of the households were contained in either detached or semidetached (two-family) houses. These buildings are generally constructed of cement blocks, bricks, or *bahareque*—a form of adobe held together with strips of wood. Of the approximately 20 percent of the families who owned or were buying homes in the barrio, about one-half were purchasing detached and half semidetached houses.

The majority of Las Crucitas residents, however, live in one of several types of *cuarterias*, or rows of connected rooms that are differentiated by their arrangement. *Cuarterias de la calle* are single rows of such rooms that generally face the street; *cuarterias de los callejones* are arranged in double rows facing each other across a narrow alleyway that may run the entire length of a block. Both types, together with other combinations of connected rooms scattered across back lots, are decidedly substandard. There is no owner-occupancy of this kind of housing. Constructed of wood or,

---

Table III-1. Type of Housing in Las Crucitas
(in percent)

Houses	32	
Single *(Casa Aislada)*		17
Double *(Casa Contigua)*		15
Rooms (Cuarterias)	68	
In row house facing street *(a la Calle)*		26
In row house on alley *(de Callejon)*		24
In house on back lot *(Casa con Cuarterias)*		18
Total	100	
Number of cases	(400)	

SOURCE: Census Sample A.

---

less frequently, *bahareque* and earthen floors, they are generally windowless with the door serving for both access and ventilation. An average of six persons and all functions of daily life are housed in the single room, sometimes with a small kitchen in the rear covered by an overhang of the tiled roof. The *cuarterias de callejones* are particularly oppressive since the dirt alleyway between the buildings that face each other is barely wide enough for a person to walk through. The alley must serve as both a sewage and waste disposal area and as a long, narrow "courtyard" for as many as 120 to 150 persons.

Table III-2 shows that not only did clear differences exist between the education of the heads of the households residing in a house and those residing in a *cuarteria*, but also between the two types of *cuarterias*. Nearly twice as many heads of households living in *cuarterias de callejones* had little or no education compared to those living in the *cuarterias* facing on a street.

The majority of the barrio's residents identified lack of water as the most serious problem facing them (Table III-3). Only 38 percent of all households had water supplied to them, and the remainder had to buy it from the more fortunate or carry it from the river or streams located at some distance downhill. When droughts are particularly acute, water must be delivered by truck. With respect to health, the source of water matters very little because the public water supply for the entire urban area is polluted. Although water should be boiled and filtered before use, 70 percent of the households in subsamples A_1 and A_2 did not take this precaution.

Other problems of the physical environment most frequently mentioned in the interviews were the poor conditions of barrio roads and poor sanitation.[2]

Table III-2.   Type of Housing, by Education of Head of Household (in percent)

Education	House	Row House Facing Street	Row House on Alley	Total
None	27	28	45	100
1-3 years	27	25	48	100
4-6 years	44	30	26	100
7 years or more	64	18	18	100
Number of cases				(400)

SOURCE: Census Sample A.

Seventeen percent of the households had private toilet facilities while 41 percent had access to latrines and other such common facilities. Forty percent, however, had no available facilities. The picture is similar with respect to other forms of sanitation. Only 30 percent of the households receive the services of a garbage truck, and, of these, two out of every three said that pickups were infrequent. Nearly one-half reported that they disposed of their garbage by finding some place for it near their house, often the street or a vacant lot. This method of waste disposal, combined with the lack of storm sewers and adequate drainage, produces major problems of sanitation about which health residents accurately complain. Following a heavy rainfall, flat areas and clogged drains (often only badly eroded ditches) fill with debris and sewage to produce both an assault on the senses and a serious challenge to health. The problems of environmental sanitation are reflected in the high rates of intestinal disorders, infectious diseases, and infant deaths. For example, estimates from pregnancy histories indicate that between one-fourth and one-third of all children conceived will not live to adolescence.

Table III-3. Identification of Problems Facing Barrio Residents (in percent)

Problems	Mentioned[a]	First Mentioned
Lack of water	53	36
Poor condition of the streets	51	21
Garbage, poor sanitation	45	15
Lack of lights	21	3
Housing, landlords	10	3
Bad environment, drunkenness	7	4
Poverty, lack of work	6	4
Little safety, no police	6	2
Poor health services	2	0
Other problems	7	2
No problems	6	6
No answer, don't know	5	5
Number of cases		(400)

SOURCE: Census Sample A.

[a] Percentages total more than 100 percent because multiple answers were given.

In summary, a picture of a hostile physical environment in Las Crucitas emerges. The picture is still incomplete, however, since the residents of Las Crucitas live in a *social* as well as a physical environment. Judgments about the physical environment, especially housing, are made in a social context. For example, the fact that only 10 percent of the respondents mentioned housing (or landlords) as a major problem facing them suggests that such judgments are strongly influenced by an awareness of the quality of housing available elsewhere in Honduras. As bad as housing (or other conditions) in Las Crucitas may be, the housing elsewhere is viewed as worse or more expensive. Despite the indicators revealing the population to be one of low status, it is not at the bottom of the urban social and economic structure.

There are other indicators that the difficulties of physical environment are not independent of social factors. The lack of services in Las Crucitas that many urban residents in Tegucigalpa take for granted is not only the result of physical obstacles to their construction, but is also due to economic difficulties and the failure of many landlords to provide the basic services required by urban authorities. Neglect, apathy, and a sense of powerlessness on the part of barrio dwellers combine to keep the situation from being improved. One resident of Las Crucitas expressed the sentiments and plight of many:

> And here, what is one to do? Everyone here is poor. If we had leaders who would help in something—but here it is not even worth the effort.

Social Environment

An examination of Table III-3 shows a problem unrelated to physical environment does not appear until fifth in the order of frequency mentioned. Even then the problem mentioned, "housing and landlords," is a mixture of physical and social problems. Less than 17 percent of all responses concerned such social problems as poverty, drunkenness, lack of employment, and public safety. Only four respondents commented on health services, and no one mentioned overcrowding, rapid growth, or other topics of demographic interest.

Responses, however, reflected the context of the questions, the amount of interview rapport, and similar factors. In the longer, semi-structured interviews, respondents were asked to cite "an important topic of conversation between husband and wife" and "an important step or decision affecting the family during the previous twelve months" (Table III-4). While such matters as poverty, employment, and health did appear as topics of considerable concern and thereby reflected the social conditions in the barrio, these matters tended to be expressed as problems related specifically to the individual or the family. Such reflections of the social ambience in the barrio as social control and public safety, general levels of poverty, and common problems of health were missing. Health, for example, was discussed in the context of the threat to the respondent's income if he were ill or the need for major expenditure in connection with a child's illness. It is seldom presented in terms of the prevalence of disease or high levels of infant mortality. (This pattern is found in other studies of Latin American urban areas.[3]) Residents of the barrio seemed to relate to their social environment in only the most particularistic of ways.

If so, then one would expect to find few indications of solidarity or even social interaction among residents in the barrio. Such an

Table III-4.   Topics of Discussion and Decision
among Families (in percent)

An Important Topic of Conversation between Husband and Wife	Reported by Husband	Reported by Wife
Poverty	49	17
Health	10	4
Leaving barrio	10	7
Children's school	10	13
Everyday matters, other	21	59
Total	100	100
Important Decision affecting Family in Past Twelve Months		
Health	49	4
Housing	26	30
Work	8	8
Other a	11	38
No decision	6	20
Total	100	100
Number of cases	(53)b	(212)

a Including children, education, a major purchase, and household matters.
b Subsample A_1. Females are from the combined subsamples A_1 and A_2.

expectation may seem implausible in a situation of high population density and close living arrangements, despite the high migration that characterizes the barrio. Nevertheless, the predictions of low solidarity and interaction are borne out by the research findings. For example, of the 400 men and women interviewed in Sample A, only 9 percent belonged to any organization. These included two "barrio improvement" organizations—"Patronato El Pastel" and the "Patronato Centro de Salud"; church organizations; athletic or social clubs; Alcoholics Anonymous; and labor organizations.

Further, only 19 percent of the males said that they received aid from their neighbors. When asked why, nearly one-half said that no one helps others because the people in the barrio are unfriendly. Similarly, only 11 percent reported that they had ever been given credit by barrio businessmen.

Women in Sample B were asked whom they visited frequently among friends, relatives, and neighbors (Table III-5). Since most of these women spend their day near home, it is surprising to discover that less than 25 percent frequently visited with neighbors and only about one-third had neighbors come to visit them. In contrast, the responses for frequent visits with relatives, including parents, were 54 and 70 percent, respectively.

Additional evidence of this pattern was obtained in a series of intensive interviews with twenty persons who had lived in the barrio for a long period of time, generally over fifteen years. Only seven of the families knew more than six other families in the barrio, seven knew between three and six other families, and six did not know

Table III-5.   Frequent Visits, by Relationship
            (in percent)

Relationship	Go to Visit Frequently	Come to Visit Frequently
No one	37	26
Parents	17	17
Other relatives	37	53
Close personal friends	15	18
Neighbors	23	35
Friends outside the barrio	9	9
Acquaintances from work	3	4
Others	3	—

Source: Census Sample B.

any other families in Las Crucitas despite the fact that they had lived there for an average of twenty years! In part, these long-term residents are set off from the other barrio residents by their older age and higher economic status, not to mention the absence of a propensity to move.[4] But the rapid turnover leaves only those with some residential permanence with the possibility for developing social networks in the barrio. If such networks are weak in this group, they are even weaker in the barrio in general.

Not only were social solidarity and interaction low in Las Crucitas, but suspicion and even hostility appeared to prevail. What does this mean for program planning? The comments of one man who had recently moved between barrios within the study area summarize the difficulties and feelings of many:

> When I lived in Colonia Obrera, the people were very bad and there was a lot of fighting going on. I did not like that and we decided to move to this barrio. I was sick also and since I had no money I could not see a doctor and decided to be cured at home, with homemade medicines . . . and I do not like the company of others. [With respect to the future] I don't know because that changes all the time. God decides it, sometimes for better; others for the worse.

Programs to effect change in the barrios, be it the construction of better sanitation services or a reduction in the birth rate, must take account of this man and others like him.

In addition, the initiative for change must come from persons or agencies from outside of the barrio. The great majority of barrio residents not only did not participate in organizations, but they were without effective leadership for organizing change. In the interviews with subsamples A_1 and A_2, only 15 percent could name a community leader. An additional 20 percent said that a few persons were qualified to be leaders but did not assert themselves. Fifty percent, however, said that no one in the barrio was qualified to be a leader. Even if a leader tried to emerge from within the barrio, it seems likely that few persons would recognize him.

The record of efforts to develop community interest and support in barrio projects both reflects this situation and contributes to it. The lack of community support for various projects has caused them to fail with regularity, and, in turn, the failures have discouraged others from beginning new programs or even participating in them. The unavailability of water, poor streets, lack of lights, and poor sanitation have long been defined as the major barrio problems whose solutions require decisions by public agencies and the absentee landlords who control much of the land. But local institutions and barrio leaders have never been able to cause the necessary decisions to be made. This inability has resulted in resentment and suspicion among the people of Las Crucitas.

The lack of interaction in the barrio has one immediate implication for family planning programs. There are several possible procedures for informing and motivating a community about family planning. One approach stresses a communications campaign to reach appropriate individuals in the barrio directly; another reaches the target population indirectly through opinion leaders and those friends and neighbors with whom intimate matters can be discussed. Proponents of the second procedure contend that the discussion of family planning and related topics with others establishes their legitimacy and reinforces favorable opinions towards them, leading to possible action. Each approach has been successful in experimental situations, but, of the two, only the direct approach could have worked in a barrio where suspicion of neighbors and low social solidarity were widely present.[5]

Possibly the mass communications campaign that was conducted in Las Crucitas will stimulate only a certain percentage of the total group in need of birth control services to seek them. Later it may be necessary to employ the other procedure to pass a threshold at which rates of clinic attendance or other measures of family planning use are beginning to level off. But in the area of fertility control, that time is not the present in urban Honduras.

Demographic Features

Regardless of the method of measurement, fertility in Las Crucitas cannot be described in any way other than *extremely high*. The pyramid shown in Figure III-1 is a graphic representation of the population's age and sex composition and reflects the interaction of fertility, mortality, and migration. It shows that nearly one-half of the barrio population is under fifteen years of age. Not only does this reflect the very high fertility levels of the population, but it emphasizes the great pressure that such levels of fertility place on existing and future services. For example, there are more than 3,300 children in Las Crucitas[6] below the age of ten years who, given the high incidence of infectious and intestinal diseases, will frequently need medical attention.

Although conventional measures of fertility are difficult to obtain from survey data, and Honduras does not have a well-developed vi-

Figure III-1.   Las Crucitas Population Pyramid, 1968

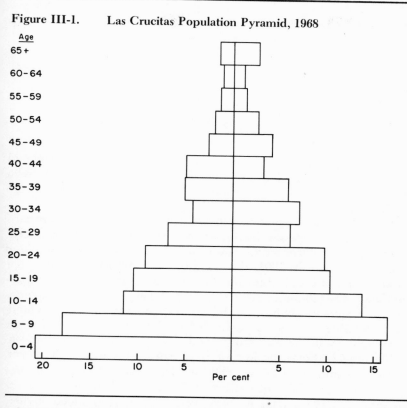

tal registration system, it is important to know how the fertility of Las Crucitas compares with that of the entire Honduran population, especially its urban component. While child-woman ratios (number of children 0– 4 years of age per 1,000 women of the reproductive ages, 15— 44 years) provide only a crude measure, they facilitate comparison with the 1961 Honduran census.

Despite the time differences in the comparisons, one can see in Table III-6 that fertility is very high in Las Crucitas. It is twice that of the urban population of the Department of Francisco Morazan, not only the most heavily urban of the Departments in Honduras, but the one containing Tegucigalpa-Comayaguela.

Since Tegucigalpa-Comayaguela represents 96 percent of the total *urban* population of Francisco Morazan, the comparison is in fact between the child-woman ratio for the barrio in 1968 and the city that contains it in 1961. The comparison is distorted somewhat by

Table III-6.   Child-Woman Ratios for Las Crucitas,
                1968, and Other Honduran
                Populations, 1961

	Urban	Rural	Total
Las Crucitas	—	—	865
Honduras	730	995	925
Francisco Morazan	359	485	418

this seven-year difference: the reported infant mortality declined substantially in the period, and the number of children born who lived long enough to be enumerated in either the census or the sample increased.[7]

Fertility for Las Crucitas may be even higher than these comparisons suggest. The age-sex figures show a substantial underenumeration of female children in the age group 0 − 4 years when compared to the 1961 census. In 1961, the sex ratio was 102 for the entire nation and for Francisco Morazan. For the 1968 sample, the comparable figure was 133 males per 100 females.[8] The most likely explanation is a systematic failure by barrio respondents to report young girls as members of their households.[9] Differential migration by sex is very unlikely in this age group, and the sex ratios fall within reasonable ranges above the age of five years. This means, however, that had the number of female children been counted in the same ratio as reported in the 1961 census of Honduras, then the child-woman ratio in Las Crucitas in 1968 would have been much higher, possibly reaching 974, excluding the effects of infant mortality.

The total fertility rate (TFR), considered to be the best cross-sectional measure of fertility, can also be calculated for Las Crucitas. This rate estimates the number of children women would have if they all went through their reproductive ages exposed to the pattern of age-specific fertility in effect at a particular time.[10] If the TFR is slightly over 2.0 per woman (or 2,000 per 1,000 women),[11] then the population is not growing, but replacing itself. Values greatly exceeding 2.0, however, indicate that the population is growing rapidly. Estimates by the United Nations for Honduras indicate that the total fertility rate is approximately 6.3—one of the highest in the world.[12] (Comparable figures, for example, for Sweden and Puerto Rico are 2.3 and 4.9, respectively.) The total fertility rate for Las Crucitas in 1967 was still higher—about 7.7. This means that if present levels of fertility in Las Crucitas continue, women could have averaged seven or eight live births as they completed their reproductive span. With present levels of foetal loss, this would require an average of more than nine pregnancies,

These figures, however, are averages for all women who are in the reproductive ages. If the analysis is restricted to women aged 15 — 44 years of proven fertility (i.e., one or more children and currently mated), the total fertility rate rises to over ten. Since these are the women who are most immediately in need of family planning services, much of the discussion of fertility that follows will focus on them.

Nevertheless, the other group, largely women not living in a current marital union, could cause fertility rates to climb if various social changes were to occur.[13] At the time of the study, this group included 46 percent of the women aged 15 — 44 years in Las Crucitas. Of these, nearly one-half had had a previous union and were widowed or separated. An additional 19 percent were women who had not had a previous union, marital or otherwise, but were over the age of 20, by which time four-fifths of all women in Las Crucitas have entered their first union. The remaining 36 percent were unmarried girls under 20 who collectively represented nearly one out of every six women in the reproductive ages.

While some of the women in the group without spouses have had children and their TFR was higher than that for the United States in 1968, this category basically represents a demographic Democles sword. Exposure to risk of pregnancy begins early in the barrio, with 10 percent of the women entering their first union before age 15 and 80 percent before age 20. But this exposure is interrupted by time spent between the end of one such union and the beginning of another. About 40 percent of the currently mated women have had more than one union, and one-half of them had already entered their second union by age 20. The figures for the group presently without husbands or partners is much higher. A change in the social and economic situation of Las Crucitas leading to greater family stability, other things equal, could drive the already high rates of fertility upwards.

To summarize, fertility is extremely high, much higher even than that for urban Honduras in general. Second, modest evidence suggests that fertility in Las Crucitas may have increased in the past few years. Third, the measures may be underestimating present levels of fertility since female children (and most likely births as well) are underenumerated. Finally, potential exists for further increases in fertility. Improved health conditions, leading to less foetal loss and lower rates of maternal mortality, could contribute to increased fertility as could reductions in the amount of reproductive time lost between unions.

Migration

Viewed in combination, Tables III-7 and III-8 indicate that the great majority of heads of households were born in the *campo*. Only 16 percent were born in Tegucigalpa-Comayaguela, and nearly 60 percent were born in rural areas or communities with less than 1,000 population at the time of the 1961 census. Migrants to the capital did not move far, however. The largest group came from the Department of Francisco Morazan in which the capital city is located, and one-half of the rest came from the departments of El Paraiso,

---

Table III-7.   Birthplace of Heads of Households

Department of Birth	Percent	
Francisco Morazan	56	
Capital		16
Elsewhere		40
Choluteca	8	
La Paz	8	
El Paraiso	7	
Elsewhere in Honduras	17	
Foreign born	4	
Information not available	1	
Total	100	
Population of Birthplace		
Rural	59	
1,000-2,499	7	
2,500-4,999	7	
5,000-9,999	5	
10,000-49,999	3	
More than 50,000	16	
Information not available	4	
Total	100	
Number of cases	(400)	

SOURCE: Census Sample A.

Choluteca, and La Paz—all of which are contiguous to Francisco Morazan.

The principal reasons for migration reported by male household heads who had migrated were economic conditions and opportunities for work (60 percent). These were perceived as poor in the rural area and better in the city. Other major reasons included family considerations (15 percent) and access to education and other predominantly urban services (10 percent). Their reasons for moving to Tegucigalpa rather than some other urban center, however, were motivated less by anticipated employment opportunities (12 percent) than they were by the related factors of proximity (31 percent) and the presence of family already in the city (43 percent).

For the male and female heads of households who were not born in the city, the dates of their arrival in Tegucigalpa were rather evenly spread over the past twenty-five years. Seventeen percent arrived since 1965, and approximately equivalent proportions arrived in each of four preceding five-year periods. Arrival in the study area, however, is much more concentrated in the period since 1965.

Table III-8.   Arrival of Heads of Households in Las Crucitas and Tegucigalpa (in percent)

Arrival in Tegucigalpa		Arrival in Las Crucitas	
Before 1929	3		
1930-1939	9		
1940-1944	6		
1944-1949	10		
1950-1954	10	Before 1954	9
1955-1959	13	1954-1959	11
1960-1964	15	1960-1964	27
1965	3	1965	6
1966	5	1966	11
1967	6	1967	16
1968[a]	3	1968[a]	21
Born in city	16	Born in barrio	1
No answer	2	No answer	1
Total	100	Total	100
Number of cases	(400)	Number of cases	(400)

SOURCE: Census Sample A.

[a]A few months before the interview.

Over one-half of the heads of households (and generally their families) had moved to Las Crucitas since that time. Part of this concen-
tration is the result of the construction of new housing, but most of
it is a reflection of the great frequency of migration by many of the
barrio's residents. Migration histories indicate that about 25 percent
of the heads of households had migrated directly to Las Crucitas
from the *campo*, while the rest had lived in other parts of the city.
Table III-8, which permits a comparison of dates of arrival in the
city and in the barrio, suggests that many residents of Las Crucitas
are exposed to a minimum of several years of residence in Tegucigalpa before moving to their present barrio of residence. Household

---

Table III-9.   Mean Number of Live Births, by Age and Migration Status

Present Age of Woman	Born in City	Migrated before 1949	Migrated between 1950 and 1968
15-24	2.3	—	2.3
25-34	3.8	5.6	4.4
35-44	5.3	6.2	6.2
Number of cases	(33)	(39)	(135)

SOURCE: Combined subsamples A_1 and A_2.

Table III-10.   Female Attitudes toward Family Planning, by Population of Birthplace (in percent)

Population of Birthplace	Attitude toward Family Planning			Number of Cases
	Uses	Approves But Does Not Use	Opposes	
Rural	20	62	18	(112)
1,000-2,499	22	50	28	(18)
2,500-4,999	26	58	16	(19)
5,000-9,999	38	50	12	(16)
10,000-49,999	28	36	36	(11)
More than 50,000	50	44	6	(32)
All Women	27	56	18	(208)

SOURCE: Combined subsamples A_1 and A_2.

heads had moved an average of three times within the city, and about one in seven have moved five or more times. About 15 percent of the respondents had moved at least once within the four-barrio study area.

The lack of organization and leadership and the suspicion and detachment that characterize social relationships are in part consequences of this rapid turnover of the population. While migration poses serious problems for the planning of programs, it can be turned to advantage in localized programs, such as family planning, since the migrants can spread information throughout the city as they move.

Finally, Table III-9 suggests that migrant women over age 24 had higher fertility than those born in the city. The probable link between rural origins of women and fertility is demonstrated in Table III-10. The women who were born in Tegucigalpa were more than twice as likely to use birth control as those who migrated to the city. Similarly, opposition to family planning was considerably less frequent among women native to Tegucigalpa than among those who were born elsewhere. Partial explanation for this pattern can be found in the association between migration status and other variables displayed in Table III-11. Rural origins, socioeconomic status reflected by housing situation, and illiteracy are closely connected and in combination produce these attitudes toward family planning. Campaigns to attack high fertility must take these factors into account.

Table III-11. Housing and Literacy, by Population of Birthplace (in percent)

Population of Birthplace	Living in Cuarterias	Literate	Number of Cases
Rural	63	42	(112)
1,000-2,499	72	61	(18)
2,500-4,999	68	58	(19)
5,000-9,999	63	69	(16)
10,000-49,999	36	73	(11)
More than 50,000 (Tegucigalpa)	31	91	(32)
All Women	58	56	(208)

SOURCE: Females from subsamples A_1 and A_2.

Socioeconomic Status

One strong indicator of socioeconomic status is educational attainment. Table III-12 presents the last year of school attended by the heads of households interviewed in the census sample. Thirty-six percent had received no education, and the median year of school attended was less than two years. Predictably, more than one-half indicated they were unable to read or write.

About 40 percent of those who could not read reported that someone read to them at least once a week, but conversely, one-half of those who stated that they could read indicated they seldom or never read a newspaper.

By combining information on employment and occupation, the amount of unemployment in the barrio can be estimated. The analysis is confused by the fact that about one-half of all persons over 10 years of age made some contribution to household income, usually through part-time employment. Attention here will be restricted to the employment situation of heads of households.

Only 11 percent of household heads were unemployed at the time of interview, although an additional 6 percent were housewives who must rely on other members of the household for their support. But this information must be tempered with information on the frequen-

---

Table III-12.   Last Year of School Attendance of Heads of Households (in percent)

Last Year of School Attendance	Percent
None	36
First	6
Second	16
Third	15
Fourth	7
Fifth	5
Sixth	7
Secondary school (7-12)	4
University	2
No answer	3
Total	100
Number of cases	(400)

SOURCE: Census Sample A.

cy that persons had worked during the preceding six months. Combining both the presently employed and unemployed household heads (excluding nonworking housewives), only three-fourths had worked the entire period without interruption. Ten percent had worked three months or less, and 6 percent had not worked at all. In addition, many of those who were employed worked for only a portion of the week.[14]

The pattern of irregular work is partially explained by the low level of skills characteristic of the household heads. More than 60 percent indicated that they were sales persons or artisans and laborers. Of those working in sales, nearly all were street vendors, the proprietors of small stores, or participants in related work. In the other category, a sizable minority were tailors, shoe makers, masons, carpenters, or participants in other skilled or semi-skilled occupations; but the largest categories were those of general laborers or persons with unspecified skills. The economic situation in Las Crucitas is a combination of both unemployment and underemployment. Income is low, and, equally important, regular work is often uncertain. Both factors are important in determining the social environment of the barrio and the problems faced by families within it.

A picture emerges of a population living in a marginal situation for which high rates of fertility and migration compound the problems and present challenges to their solution. But the population is clearly not homogeneous. While most residents of Las Crucitas are of low socioeconomic status, a sizable minority have been regularly employed as professionals, "white-collar workers," or skilled artisans. Much of the housing is extremely poor, but a number of the houses are well-constructed, substantial buildings. The majority of residents had lived in the houses for less than four years, but a sizable minority had been there for many years. Even among the latter, there were some who were economically comfortable, while others were living in poverty.

The Health Center and Its Clients

The importance of providing adequate health and family planning services should be clear from the description of the barrio and its inhabitants. Difficulties with water supply and environmental sanitation that were identified by the great majority of residents as the most important problems facing the barrio are directly reflected in the high rate of infant mortality [15] and the high incidence of infectious disease and intestinal disorders.[16] Disease and poor health are part of the way of life in the barrio, and the Las Crucitas Health Center is the "first line of defense" against these conditions, both through medical care and its programs of health education. Similarly, the Health Center through its family planning clinic offers one response to problems of high fertility in the barrio. Opportunities for such service are heightened by a clear interest of many barrio residents in limiting family size.[17]

But the need for health services and their availability do not necessarily lead to their effective use. The complexity of the situation can be seen in examining problems of health in the barrio, the organization of the Las Crucitas Health Center, and knowledge and perceptions that the barrio residents have of the Health Center.

Health Problems

Despite expressed concern with environmental health problems (water, sanitation), problems of personal health were found to be infrequently discussed by residents of the barrio. Only 4 percent of the females and 9 percent of the males mentioned health as a topic of routine family discussion. (As might be expected in an area where full and regular employment is uncertain, males reported that problems of poverty and economic conditions dominate their daily family conversation.) Health became a matter of considerable concern, however, when these respondents were asked about *serious* problems that face them. One-half of the males cited a health problem as the principal family "crisis" of the preceding year requiring a major decision.[18] Poor health and illness appeared to be taken for granted and worthy of general discussion only when they developed into a crisis situation or when income was threatened. There is an orientation toward the present rather than the future in the matters of health. For many, poor health is something to be cured rather than prevented. Barrio residents accept a certain level of illness as "normal," and complaints about poor sanitation and other environmental hazards are not transformed into discussions of personal and family health. The use of unboiled water by 70 percent of the study population and the indiscriminate disposal of garbage and other waste by one-half of those interviewed underline this situation,[19] and opinions directed towards the Health Center reinforce this assessment. Table III-13 indicates that while virtually everyone interviewed knew of the Health Center, there were great differences in the awareness of services provided by it. While 56 percent men-

**Table III-13. Knowledge of Services Available at
Las Crucitas Health Center (in percent)**

Service	Mentioned[a]	First Mentioned
Sick-children clinic	56	37
Injections	38	8
Immunizations	37	8
Maternal hygiene	18	6
Milk and nutrition	17	4
Well-children clinic	13	5
Laboratory	8	1
Dental	8	1
Social services	4	1
Family planning	2	—
Sanitation services	2	—
Do not know any	36	—

SOURCE: Census Sample A.

[a]Percentages add up to more than 100 percent because of multiple responses.

tioned its services for sick children, only 13 percent mentioned that services were available for well children. (Only 2 percent mentioned that family planning services were available.) The Health Center is generally viewed as providing services for persons, particularly children, who are ill and not oriented toward persons who are "well."[20] While this view is to some extent realistic, it is also part of the general view of health as something to be confronted when it happens rather than before it can occur.

Views of the Health Center

While there are also family planning and other clinics at the San Felipe Hospital serving the population of the capital, the Health Center in Las Crucitas is much more convenient to the barrio's residents because none live farther than a ten-minute walk. But convenience must be measured in ways other than physical distance. The organization of services at the Health Center, the manner in which patients are received and treated, and the way in which patients perceive their treatment are among the factors that will determine whether persons will use its facilities, seek the same services elsewhere, or perhaps receive no services at all.

Two procedures were used to gather information on the Health Center and services to patients. First, various questions were asked about when and where various health services were sought and how the recipients felt about them;[21] and second, a member of the research group spent four weeks observing the operation of the Center in general and its family planning clinic in particular.[22]

The residents' overall view of the Health Center's delivery of health services is not highly favorable.[23] Although the doctors and nurses working in the Health Center are professionally capable, medical care is not optimally delivered in the eyes of the patients who need that care. The manner in which different services are organized and the times at which they are offered, the necessity for the doctors and the administrator to divide their time between the Las Crucitas Health Center and other health agencies in the capital, a confusing organizational structure in which the Health Center and various clinics within it are placed, shortage of equipment and materials, and the demands of a population in which ill-health is frequent are all obstacles to the optimal delivery of health care.

This assessment is substantiated by what happened when the mass communication campaign took place. Paralleling radio and other announcements on the availability of family planning services at the clinic, the services were reorganized and expanded to meet the increased demand, yet the staff and administration were essentially the same. The change in patterns of use reported below occurred because of the increased demand and was facilitated by the removal of some of the obstacles noted above.

Table III-14.   Institutions Mentioned for Health
Services (in percent)

Institution	Mentioned[a]	First Mentioned
Las Crucitas Health Center	57	27
Alonso Suazo Health Center	8	3
San Felipe Hospital	76	51
Seguro Social Hospital	18	7
Polyclinics	3	2
Private clinic, doctor	11	7
Other	5	2
No answer	2	—

[a]Percentages add up to more than 100 percent because of multiple responses.

While almost all respondents knew of the Health Center, more than 40 percent reported that they did not use it. Table III-14 reports on the institutions that were used. In those households that did use its services, 22 percent had someone visit the Center within the previous month, and more than 75 percent had gone within the past year. To extrapolate from the data on use and nonuse, more than 5 percent of the households that the Health Center serves will have direct contact with it for some kind of care within a *single* average week. Ninety percent of these visits were for medical care for children, an additional 7 percent involved mothers, and only 3 percent of the visits to the Health Center were by males or other female adults in the household. The specific reasons for the visits are presented in Table III-15. About three out of every four visits involved illness or injury, with intestinal disorders being most frequent. Only one-fifth of the visits involved preventive medical care such as a vaccination or examinations.

When those who did not use the Health Center were asked why, about one-half gave reasons not related to the health services provided (e.g., never sick, receive their care elsewhere, or had just arrived in the barrio). The remainder indicated that poor service caused them to go elsewhere. Table III-16 summarizes these responses. They coincide closely with the criticisms of the Health Center offered spontaneously by about 10 percent of all respon-

---

Table III-15. Reasons for Most Recent Visit to Health Center

Reason	Percent
Vaccination, clinical examination	18
Pre- or post-natal care	5
Family planning	—
Respiratory ailment, communicable disease	21
Intestinal disorder	28
General complaint (headaches, earaches, etc.)	18
Chronic illness	5
Injury	1
No answer	5
Total	100
Number of cases	(259)

SOURCE: Census Sample A.

Table III-16.   Reasons for Not Using the Health Center

Reason	Percent Mentioned
Not necessary, never been sick here	26
Go to other institutions	16
Just arrived, new here	7
Does not treat adults	5
Generally poor services	11
Overcrowding, long waits	10
Inconvenient hours	4
High costs of medicine	1
No medicines available	1
Other	13
No answer	7
Total	100
Number of cases	(147)

SOURCE: Census Sample A.

dents during the course of the interviews. The most frequent comment among that 10 percent concerned the long waits and crowding at the clinic (42 percent), followed by the unavailability of medicine (16 percent) or its high cost (7 percent), and poor service received (13 percent). About 20 percent of the spontaneous criticisms[24] concerned the belief that the Health Center did not treat adults.

Use of the Health Center varies with socioeconomic and migrant status. For example, only 41 percent of those with seven or more years of education but about two-thirds of those with less education used the Center. Similarly, those respondents who had arrived within the barrio during the previous six months used the services less (41 percent) than those who had been there for one or two years (62 percent) or longer (74 percent).

One-half of the respondents did not know that the Center provided family planning services.

Observation within the Center

The observations of the researcher working within the Health Center substantiated many of the criticisms voiced by residents.[25]

Heavy demand for services, for example, leads directly to the over-crowding and the long waits that residents complain about and indirectly to the manner in which patients are treated at the clinic. Although the Center opens around 6:00 A.M., patients begin arriving long before in order to secure a place in line. In the pediatric clinics and in the general adult clinic, there is a quota imposed on the number of patients to be seen in each session. Many patients have learned that they must arrive by a certain hour in order to be seen. Those who do not receive an appointment must return the next day and begin the entire procedure again. Thus, long waits for attention in crowded waiting rooms become one aspect of seeking care.

In addition, since Center personnel must screen patients in order to see those who need immediate care, well children receive a lower priority for attention than sick children. This means that such services as nutrition and family planning are assigned lower priorities by nursing aides and the medical staff, as well as by the population of the barrio.

Since even this screening procedure is often not enough to reduce the patient load, mothers with more than one child needing attention cannot have them treated at the same time, and patients are not treated if their records are not in order. On occasion, even when the number of patients that could be seen in a clinic was manageable, physicians remained idle because the patient's records could not be assembled. During a week of the observational study, one doctor spent a total of five hours waiting for additional patients to be assigned to him.

The problems involving patient records are serious in other ways. Each patient has a folder-type record that is stored by number, but often these cannot be easily found. This can lead to a delay or a denial of service. In addition, the physicians working in regular clinics at the Health Center arrive between 5:30 and 6:00 A.M., but the record room does not open until 7:00 A.M. The delay of an hour between the beginning of services and the availability of records hinders service. Further, the physical arrangement of the record center presents real difficulties. It is located in the main waiting room where patients mill around it. The high noise level makes it difficult for the record clerk and patients to converse with one another. Many persons stand for one or two hours waiting for their names to be called. If a patient happens not to hear her number called and fails to respond, she can lose her appointment with the doctor.

The pharmacy is also a major source of confusion and a cause of patient discontent. On many occasions, drugs that are supposed to be available are not. For example, on the days that the adult clinic was observed, approximately three-quarters of the drugs were crossed off the druggist's list because of their unavailability. As a result, the doctor had to send seventeen out of twenty patients treated to the San Felipe Hospital for follow-up treatment.

The evening clinic provides another example of the problems faced by the Health Center. Designed to serve emergency pediatric cases and persons who could not come during the day because of their employment, the evening clinic is instead generally required to serve the overflow of cases built up from earlier hours. The original purpose of the clinic is defeated by the heavy demands for service. What is true for the evening clinic is true for the Health Center in general. The need for medical attention within the population served by it greatly exceeds available resources. Even the manner in which the clinic personnel deal with patients can be traced partially to this situation.

Provision of family planning services is more difficult than the offering of regular health services, and all of the problems of the Health Center mentioned above would especially weaken the effective delivery of family planning services. The image of the Health Center as a place for handling the illnesses of children might to some effect deter potential clients. Having to wait for long periods on a low-priority basis and with the possibility of then being asked to return at another time might also be expected to discourage potential adopters of family planning. For persons who work, the regular Center hours might require a loss of pay if such advice was sought. The necessity to acknowledge a desire for family planning to a harried clerk in a crowded waiting room would be enough to discourage most shy women from seeking information or service. All of these situations and others are less problematic when the relief from pain or illness drives the patient to the Center.

Since the researchers did not want such administrative bottlenecks to defeat an otherwise successful mass media campaign for family planning, a program of expanded services was arranged to begin just prior to the initiation of the campaign. A greater variety and quantity of medicines and contraceptives were provided, and two doctors, two nurse's aides, and a full-time public health nurse were added to the staff. Night hours (7:00 - 9:00, five nights a week) and a Saturday morning clinic were added. Major reorganization of the Health Center was unnecessary, suggesting that the answers to many of the Health Center's problems involve the increased availability of resources to its personnel.

The Communications Campaign

The mass media experiment was designed to answer a number of questions: 1) Can a low income, poorly educated population of largely rural origin be reached by modern mass media? 2) If reached, can they comprehend the message? 3) If they comprehend the message, will they change their behavior accordingly? To answer these questions an educational campaign was carried out stressing the desirability of visiting the family planning clinic, and interviews were conducted both before and after the campaign to assess its impact.

Work on Sample B, or the "Before Campaign" Survey, began the fourth week of the project immediately following completion of the Sample A census. The women of each household in Sample B were administered a battery of questions aimed at assessing attitudes, knowledge, and practice of family planning prior to the information-al campaign. On completion of these interviews, the mass communi-cation campaign began. The first phase was over the radio stations of Tegucigalpa, followed by movies at Las Crucitas Community Center and Health Center, ending with pamphlet distribution and a sound-truck campaign in the four core barrios of Las Crucitas. At the end of the campaign in the ninth week of the study, Sample C, or the "After Campaign" Survey, was administered a questionnaire almost identical to the one administered to Sample B.

Three hundred and seventy-three ever-mated women aged 15 - 49 years were interviewed prior to the campaign and 328 following it, the loss of cases due largely to the high geographic mobility of the area's residents. Nevertheless, as measured by a number of key social and demographic characteristics, the second sample seems very similar to the first, although, of course, the individuals are different (Table III-17).

Before the Campaign

General Characteristics

High fertility is again apparent, with women aged 40 - 50 years having had close to seven live births resulting in five living children. Eighty-five percent of the women were born outside of Teguci-galpa (mainly in rural areas) and half of them worked for pay. More than five of every ten women were illiterate. Even among those who claimed they can read, just under one-half said they seldom or never read a newspaper; and among those who could not

Table III-17.   Selected Characteristics before and after the Campaign (in percent)

	Before	After
Legally married	27	25
Roman Catholic	94	94
Attend church at least monthly	57	48
Have radio in house	69	70
Education		
None	37	39
1-3 years	41	40
More than 4 years	22	21
Rent per month		
Under 11 *lempiras*	30	29
11-20 *lempiras*	38	41
More than 21 *lempiras*	32	30
Age		
15-19 years	7	7
20-24 years	14	21
25-29 years	21	18
30-34 years	23	20
35-39 years	18	17
40-44 years	14	15
45-49 years	2	3
Mean live births, by age of mother		
15-19 years	0.8	1.2
20-24 years	2.1	2.3
25-29 years	3.7	3.8
30-34 years	5.0	4.8
35-39 years	6.2	6.0
40-49 years	6.6	7.0

NOTE: "No answers" have been excluded from the bases used in calculating percentages.

read, only one-third had anyone who read a newspaper to them. But the radio presents a different picture. Not only did 70 percent of the families have their own radios, but 60 to 70 percent of all women said they listened at least three hours per day. Approximately one-quarter said they listened "practically all day long."

Over two-thirds of the women had attended their neighborhood health center, and virtually all of the others had used some other public health care center such as San Felipe Hospital. Indeed, no less than 43 percent of the sample had visited a clinic in the month previous to the interview. Very few, however, had ever used these facilities to seek family planning services. When given an opportunity to mention three kinds of services they had used, less than 2 percent mentioned family planning. Moreover, when asked what services are offered by the Health Center, only 6 percent mentioned family planning, despite the fact that a majority of the women could cite three services offered by the Center. At best, the family planning services of the clinic had very low salience for these women; at worst, such services were unknown to them.

Las Crucitas women did not want especially large families. Before the campaign, 45 percent said the ideal number of children was three or less, and over two-thirds said four or less. But one-third of the women already had more than four living children. When asked how many children they would like if they were to start their own families over again, 56 percent said three or less, and 79 percent said four or less. On the other hand, many women did not go beyond the wishful thinking stage. (Some do not even go that far—four out of every ten women had never thought about the question before the interviewer asked it.) Close to six of every ten women had never discussed the number of children they wanted with their husbands, and very few reported use of a contraceptive method. Only 4 percent were taking a contraceptive pill, 6 percent were using the IUD, and only 1 percent was using rhythm. Total ignorance of contraceptive methods is not the answer, since nearly nine of every ten women interviewed before the campaign had heard about the pill and the IUD, and all of the males interviewed knew at least one method. But *awareness* of the existence of a contraceptive does not necessarily imply *knowledge* of it, and faulty knowledge can in fact lead to negative attitudes or at least to paralyzing doubt. As phrased by two respondents:

. . .Last year we talked about that, my husband and I. I told him I knew about these medicines and he told me to look for a way to stop having children. But I'm afraid. He is also afraid but suggested the pills—he's more afraid of the coil.

. . .I'm afraid. . .they say they make you bleed and make you thin, give you pains and other things.

When directly asked whether particular methods were harmful, only one-third of the women who had heard about the pill answered negatively, and a somewhat higher proportion responded in this fashion for the IUD. The source of such beliefs is primarily gossip. (Over one-half of the women interviewed in subsamples A_1 and A_2 based their knowledge of contraception on what they had heard from a friend or neighbor and only one-third from professional sources.)

Men were somewhat more knowledgeable than their wives on family planning—but slightly more conservative: 73 percent approved of birth control as opposed to 84 percent of the wives. Among those who have never used contraceptives, the proportion who had ever discussed family planning declines from two-thirds of the women who approved contraceptives to one-fourth of those who opposed it.

Among families where it had been discussed, 10 percent of the husbands were opposed to family planning *even among couples practicing contraception.* Among non-contraceptors, only 4 percent of the wives but one-third of the husbands were opposed.

It would be difficult to ignore such opposition, since 60 percent of the women reported that they are not consulted by their husbands when an important family decision is being made, and only 6 percent make decisions independently of their husbands. It is of interest that among contraceptors the wife is much more likely to be consulted on major decisions (42 percent) than among non-contraceptors (27 percent).

Age and Education

To describe the women of Las Crucitas as if they were a single or homogeneous group is to conceal a great deal of internal variation that may be of great importance for the delineation of target groups. Next to sex, the social characteristics that are possibly the most powerful predictors of human behavior are age and education; age both because it is closely linked to fertility and other biological changes and because attitudes are also profoundly influenced by it; education because it immensely increases the individual's potential for influencing and being influenced by the social environment. Because of various generational differences in access to formal schooling, age and education in most underdeveloped areas are strongly related. The sample is no exception.[26] The proportion of women who had never gone to school is only 13 percent among the very young women, but rises to a majority of the women over 40.

The sample has been divided into roughly equal numbers of "young" women (under 30 years of age) and "older" women (30 years

Table III-18. Selected Social and Demographic Characteristics, by Age and Education

	Young Women		Older Women	
	No Education	Some Education	No Education	Some Education
Percent with monthly rent over 20 lempiras	9	32	22	41
Percent with radio	62	73	61	78
Percent who listen to radio more than 3 hours daily	64	74	66	74
Percent who attend church at least once per month	40	46	48	54
Mean live births	3.5	2.4	6.2	5.6
Mean living children	2.8	2.0	4.6	4.5
Dead children per 1,000 live births	149	102	252	195
Number of cases	(42)	(107)	(88)	(91)

and over). These groups of women are subdivided into those who had never been to school and those who had had some schooling, however little. Table III-18 shows that both characteristics are related to economic status as measured by rent—the older and better educated being more "prosperous." The older women were also somewhat more likely to have a radio; but as to listening, the differences by age disappear and the differences by education narrow. The older and better educated also attended church more frequently, but again, the differences are not very great.

Attitudes toward ideal family size indicate a slight tendency for the better educated and a marked tendency for the younger women to choose smaller families (Table III-19). While this could reflect some rationalization on the part of the older women with larger families, it may also reflect a generational change; for it is evident that when asked whether or not they want more children, the older women showed no reluctance to say "no"—indeed, nine out of every ten said so. (Less-educated women were especially likely to want no more children—reflecting perhaps an acute perception of their own situations *vis-a-vis* children, despite an *ideal* slightly larger than the better educated.) The younger women, moreover, were more likely to report having thought about the number of children they wanted

**Table III-19.   Selected Family Planning Characteristics,
by Age and Education (in percent)**

	Young Women		Older Women	
	No Education	Some Education	No Education	Some Education
Ideal number of children				
3 or fewer	72	78	54	63
Want no more children	82	69	97	85
Thought about ideal number of children	86	85	68	77
Discussed desired number with spouse	52	52	24	33
Ever used birth control	31	38	17	38
Currently using birth control	24	25	14	32

and to have discussed it with their husbands, although the possibility of poorer recall on the part of the older women must be considered. Especially consistent with the hypothesis of generational change is the fact that the younger women were *already* ahead of the older women in contraceptive experience, 36 percent of them having used some method as opposed to 28 percent of the older women.

However, the uneducated were less likely to have used a contraceptive method, especially among the older generation of women. In sum, age and education were related to both attitudes and behavior, but age appears somewhat more important. This is not surprising, since the degree of variation in education is small. None of the women ever attended a university, and only 4 percent ever attended a secondary school.

Thus, a picture of the target population shows a very poor, uneducated group of high fertility women interested in limiting their fertility but not so interested or so knowledgeable as to practice much effective family planning on their own. On the other hand, they live in a compact urban neighborhood with a family planning clinic within walking distance. It would be an ideal challenge for an educational program to get them to make that walk.

The Campaign
A variety of means were employed to encourage the population to visit the family planning center—radio spot announcements, a sound truck with a nurse, pamphlets, and film.

Radio

Twenty spot announcements (fifteen to thirty seconds) were prepared in collaboration with local experts. The announcements were designed to increase clinic attendance generally, but specifically to boost attendance at the family planning clinics of Las Crucitas and San Felipe Hospital. The announcements were recorded locally, ten using a male and ten a female announcer. The seven radio stations most popular in Las Crucitas (as determined in the survey) broadcasted the "spots" each weekday for five weeks. To a background of popular music, one of four basic themes was covered in each "spot": 1) family planning services, nine announcements; 2) pre-natal or post-natal services, four announcements; 3) public health education, six announcements; 4) general services of clinic, one announcement. Illustrations of the "spots" in the three major categories are given below:

Family Planning

Parents, if you want to have only the number of children you can support, go to the family planning clinics located at San Felipe Hospital and the Las Crucitas Health Center, where the doctors will help you find a sure means without harm to your health.

More than 8,000 Honduran couples have received the benefits of the family planning clinics located in the San Felipe Hospital and the Las Crucitas Health Center, where the medical specialists will help you, free of charge.

Pre-Natal and Post-Natal Services

Madam, after having a child, visit your Health Center every three months for an examination. The doctors and nurses will help to ensure the good health of yourself and your child.

Madam, if you are expecting a baby, visit the doctor at the Las Crucitas Health Center for an examination and to ensure a healthy birth.

Public Health Education

Parents, do you know about the biggest enemies of children. Tiny animals called microbes are the biggest cause of illness. Send your family for vaccinations to Las Crucitas and Alonso Suazo Health Centers.

Madam, if you boil water for at least five minutes, you will have a healthy family. Unboiled water is a carrier of parasites. A little prevention will bring good health.

Sound Truck

The same spot announcements were also utilized by a sound truck in Las Crucitas. Each weekday over a two-week period the truck moved around the area for two hours in the morning and two hours in the afternoon. At each street corner stop a nurse inside the truck invited people to come up to the truck and ask questions about health and family planning.

Pamphlets

Three different pamphlets were distributed on two different occasions to all households (at least in theory) in Las Crucitas. The pamphlets were supplied by the Honduran Family Planning Association and dealt with specific methods of family planning. Interviewers who delivered the pamphlets were instructed to give a brief explanation of the nature and purpose of the pamphlets.

Film

Five film showings were held in Las Crucitas barrios. Each showing consisted of a commercial feature film considered popular with area residents and two documentary films, one on public health and one on family planning.[27] A total of about 450 adults and teenagers attended, about one-half of them women.

After the Campaign

There is little doubt that virtually all of the women of Las Crucitas were reached by one educational medium or another. No less than 79 percent of the after sample reported having heard about the Health Center over the radio. Exposure to the sound truck was equally impressive, with nine out of every ten women having heard the publicity. About three-quarters heard both the radio and the sound truck, and only 4 percent heard neither.[28] The data on radio listening are also quite consistent with those on exposure to the message. Fifty-five percent of the women who seldom listened to the radio, but 84 percent of those who listened three to four hours a day and 94 percent of those who listened "all day" reported having heard the broadcast. Since most women listened at least three hours per day, it is clear why most of them were reached. Thus, the crucial first step of the mass media campaign was achieved to a degree rarely realized in short-term programs—*virtually the entire target population was reached.*

Exposure to the message is a necessary but not sufficient cause for action since the message could be misunderstood or immediately forgotten. When asked what the radio or sound truck said, only 12 percent remembered nothing and another 13 percent mentioned matters (some of them correct) other than family planning. *Thus, about three-quarters mentioned that the message concerned family planning.* Furthermore, just under three-quarters mentioned spontaneously that they remembered being urged to attend Las Crucitas or San Felipe. It is possible that important parts of the message were missed. For example, when women who remembered hearing the message were asked what the radio said about not having more children, over one-half could offer nothing more specific. A similar proportion could remember no further details about the loudspeaker's message. Nevertheless, most women heard the message and understood its general point.

The respondents were apparently not offended by receiving education on family planning. In answer to the question, "Do you think it is good to receive birth control information?" 94 percent replied in the affirmative; and when asked specifically about various means, about eight of every ten approved the radio, the loudspeaker, pamphlets, movies, and talks. More than nine of every ten approved of home visits, and a similar proportion approved of physicians or nurses giving birth control information. When asked which of these various means they regarded as *most* acceptable, almost one-half chose the doctor or nurse, and another quarter chose the home visit technique.

The crucial question is the extent to which attitudes, knowledge, and behavior were affected. The first way of assessing this possible influence is to compare responses before and after the campaign.

Knowledge

There is a marked increase—nearly fivefold—in the proportion of women who mentioned family planning as one of the services offered by Las Crucitas Health Center (Table III-20). Thus the campaign probably had a decided impact in increasing the salience of this service. Since virtually all women knew about family planning before the campaign, with close to 90 percent having heard about the most up-to-date methods, little measurable impact on specific contraceptive knowledge was anticipated. Moreover, the radio carried no information on contraceptive means, and the sound truck provided little more. Only the pamphlets carried information on methods themselves. Of course, women who attended the clinic as a result of the campaign might be expected to become more knowledgeable, but not in ways that were measured—in other words, whether or not the respondent had "heard of" various methods. The surprising finding from the first part of the table is not the insubstantial increase in knowledge of modern methods, but the apparent deterioration in knowledge of conventional methods. The same trend occurs for other methods not shown on the table—withdrawal, sterilization, and rhythm.

In view of the high degree of consistency between the two surveys on questions of fact (age, education, fertility, etc.), the possibility of overall interviewer cheating is unlikely. However, an interviewer-by-interviewer examination of responses on knowledge of methods reveals that some interviewers had especially high rates of

Table III-20.   Knowledge, Attitudes, and Practice of Birth Control before and after the Campaign (in percent)

Knowledge	Before Sample	After Sample	Significance at .05
Mentioned family planning as a service of Las Crucitas Health Center	6	29	S
Heard of pill	90	91	NS
Heard of IUD	87	92	S
Heard of douche	53	20	S
Heard of condom	64	43	S
Attitudes			
Would prefer 0-3 children	56	65	S
Want no more children	63	78	S
Ever thought about desired number of children	58	79	S
Practice			
Ever sought family planning advice from health center	2	8	S
Ever visited Las Crucitas Health Center	48	62	S
Currently using birth control	19	24	NS
Current users who have used method less than one month[a]	3	18	S
Currently using pill	4	12	S
Currently using IUD	6	5	NS
Number of cases	(373)	(328)	

[a]Based on current users only, 71 cases in before sample and 78 in after sample.

reported ignorance of classical methods of contraception. Another possibility is that the campaign itself may have made people less confident about their knowledge of contraception or less willing to try to impress an interviewer with their knowledge. It may well have increased their critical abilities. Further, since those who went to the clinic were given information on the IUD and pills, other methods may have been depreciated, consciously or unconsciously. The reluctant opinion of the researchers, however, is that some interviewers were guilty of careless interviewing in the after survey.

Attitudes

On all three attitude items—ideal number of children, desire for more children, and whether there had been previous thought about number of children—there were substantial shifts after the campaign. Probably the campaign activated thought about the topic and intensified the degree of interest in small families—an interest essentially present prior to the educational program.

Behavior

It should be recalled that the "after" interviews were started the day following the close of the month-long radio campaign and only a few days after the close of the two-week sound truck campaign. Respondents had not had a great deal of time to alter their behavior, and, as judged by the overall percentage currently practicing birth control, the contribution of the campaign was not profound. Nevertheless, the possible impact on clinic attendance and use of the pill is not inconsiderable, given the time considerations. For example, although use of the IUD showed no change,[29] the proportion of current users of the pill tripled, and the proportion of current users who adopted family planning in the preceding month increased over four times. (Of course, the absolute levels were so low in the earlier survey that the significance of these apparently enormous increases should not be over-emphasized.)

Exposure to the campaign may have been responsible for many of the changes, as is indicated from Table III-21 where the degree to which the campaign message was recalled is related to some of the measures of effect. In most instances, and especially with regard to communications behavior (talking to husband or to others), the better the memory of the campaign message, the more favorable are knowledge and behavior with respect to family planning. Attitudes show little relation other than intention to use birth control. However, memory is related to age and education, with twice as

Table III-21.   Measures of Possible Campaign Effect,
by Memory of Campaign Message (in percent)

	Poor Memory	Good Memory	Significance at .05
Knowledge			
Heard of pill	87	93	S
Heard of IUD	88	94	S
Heard of condom	34	48	S
Attitudes			
Ideal number of children 3 or fewer	67	66	NS
Want no more children	85	81	NS
Ever thought about desired number of children	75	81	NS
Planning to practice birth control (among those not practicing)	45	65	S
Practice			
Discussed ideal family size with husband	18	54	S
Talked more about birth control since campaign	57	80	S
Ever used birth control	27	35	NS

NOTE: Those who remembered nothing of the campaign, or only one aspect of the message (e.g., where to go but not what for), were classified as having a "poor memory." Those who remembered at least two of the three ingredients (where, what, and why) were classified as has having a "good memory." One hundred twenty-three cases fell in the former, and 205 in the latter category. "No answers" have been excluded from the bases.

high a proportion of the older uneducated women failing to recall the message as the younger, better educated women (Table III-22).

Age and education, in turn, are related to the effect measures, as anticipated from the earlier analysis. Consequently, in Table III-23 these characteristics are held constant in broad categories as before, and the memory of the message is varied.

Memory of the campaign is related to most of the variables, holding age and education constant. The degree of discussion, both with husbands and others, is markedly related. Most young women, if they remembered the campaign message, were likely to have discussed the desired number of children with their husbands; most young

Table III-22.   Percent with Poor Memory of Message,
by Age and Education

	Young Women	Older Women	Total
No education	31	53	46
Some education	24	41	32
Total	26	47	

NOTE: Differences by age are significant at the .05 level;
differences by education are not.

women who did not recall the message had not. Closely related to this finding is the fourth part of Table III-23, indicating intention to practice family planning. If a woman was under 30 years of age and recalled the campaign message, she was almost certain to plan to use birth control (about 70 percent) if she was not already using it. Since the younger women were also much more likely to remember the message, they seem to be the ideal target groups. When this is added to the fact that changes in their fertility would have much more influence on national trends of fertility than would alterations in the fertility patterns of older women, an important conclusion emerges: *the group most important to reach, in other words, young women of relatively low parity, is not only the most "reachable" but also the most "teachable."*

Another important measure of campaign effect is clinic attendance. Figure III-2 indicates that in Las Crucitas, new admissions for the first five months of 1968 averaged between five and six per week. They rose to eleven in June (possibly as a result of personnel changes) and stayed close to that level for July. The campaign began on July 22, and increased case loads became apparent in the second week of the campaign (July 29 — August 3). During the month of August the high level established in the two preceding months tripled, reaching a level about seven times that of the first five months of the year. In the remaining months of the year there was a decline, but not to the earlier levels of the year.[30]

Moreover, there is also a decided increase in old patients, who averaged about fifty per month in the two months preceding the campaign. August showed a 50 percent increase over July, and September a comparable increase over August; by November, the case load of old patients was between three and four times that just prior to the campaign. A good share of these old patients probably represent the increased number of new admissions checking back a month later. However, at the very least the data show that the pa-

Table III-23.   Measures of Possible Campaign Effect,
by Memory of Campaign Message, Age,
and Education (in percent)

	Poor Memory	Good Memory	Total
Talked more about birth control since campaign			
Young women			
No education	62	75	70
Some education	64	80	76
Older women			
No education	50	76	63
Some education	59	86	76
Discussed ideal number of children with husband			
Young women			
No education	31	62	52
Some education	27	60	52
Older women			
No education	14	37	24
Some education	11	50	33
Have ever used birth control			
Young women			
No education	31	31	31
Some education	31	41	38
Older women			
No education	13	22	17
Some education	41	37	38

tients attending as the result of radio are not "curiosity seekers" of especially weak motivation but are at least as liable to return to the clinic as pre-campaign cases.

The data from San Felipe are not nearly so impressive. Although a peak number of cases also occurs in the month of August, the level is only 16 percent higher than the two months preceding the campaign and 38 percent higher than the average of the first five months of the year. Several explanations for the difference between clinics may be advanced. First, only Las Crucitas residents were exposed to the sound truck, pamphlets, and film. Most of the areas served by San Felipe received only the radio announcements.

	Poor Memory	Good Memory	Total
Planning to use birth control			
(among those not using)			
Young Women			
No education	60	71	68
Some education	55	76	71
Older women			
No education	43	44	43
Some education	35	62	52
Attended Las Crucitas Health Center			
Young women			
No education	54	66	62
Some education	65	60	62
Older women			
No education	55	65	60
Some education	59	69	65
Number of cases [a]			
Young women			
No education	(13)	(29)	(42)
Some education	(26)	(81)	(107)
Older women			
No education	(47)	(41)	(88)
Some education	(37)	(54)	(91)

[a] "No answers" have been deducted from the bases before percentaging.

Second, while services remained the same during the campaign at San Felipe, they were improved at Las Crucitas[31]—clinic time and medical personnel were increased. Third, the San Felipe clinic is large, efficient, and has a post-partum program in which social workers encourage maternity ward cases to visit the clinic. It is impossible to unravel how much each of these factors contributed to the greater responsiveness of the Las Crucitas community.

Additional evidence suggests that the impact of sound trucks, pamphlets, and films may not have been so great as that of radio. From the beginning of the campaign a special interview involving three questions was given to new cases entering the clinics to determine what had attracted them. They were first asked: "From whom or how did you learn about this family planning clinic?" (Table III-24).

During the major share of the four-week campaign, about one-third of Las Crucitas' new cases mentioned relatives or friends as their source of information, over one-half mentioned the radio, and over one-fourth a nurse or doctor. Toward the end of the campaign and in the weeks following it, the radio and sound truck increased markedly in influence, while relatives and friends declined in importance. Pamphlets, films, and home visitors were scarcely mentioned at all.

San Felipe cases showed smaller proportions of radio mentions, and there was little change over time except in the decline in

Figure III-2.   First Admissions per Week to Las Crucitas and San Felipe, by Month of Admission, 1968

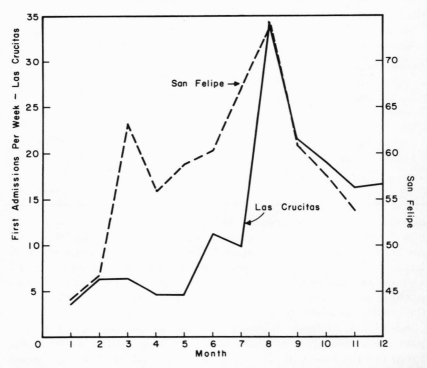

friends and relatives as sources of information. In marked contrast to Las Crucitas was the greater influence of social workers and of friends and neighbors.

These were, however, spontaneous responses. To make sure that the respondents were not overlooking other possible sources of information, a list of sources of information was read to the new patients. In each case they were asked whether or not they had heard about the clinic from this source. The procedure increased the proportion of women who mentioned radio—by eight percentage points in Las Crucitas, but by thirty-six percentage points in San Felipe. *None of the other sources showed any significant change.*

Another evidence of the superior drawing power of the radio is evidenced by the fact that most of the new admissions to Las Crucitas are from *outside* the core area. Only 28 percent of the first ninety-four new cases were from the four barrios in which the sound-truck and pamphlet campaign were conducted. Another 30 percent were from adjacent barrios, but the balance, nearly one-half of the cases, were from outside the neighborhood altogether.[32] In short, the apparent inconsistency between the modest increases in clinic attendance observed in the "before" and "after" samples and

Table III-24. **Source of Information on Family Planning Clinic for First Admissions, by Clinic and Weeks since Start of Campaign**

Source of Information	Las Crucitas			San Felipe		
	First Three Weeks	Second Three Weeks	Total	First Three Weeks	Second Three Weeks	Total
Radio	56	68	63	30	36	32
Nurse or doctor	28	30	24	37	40	38
Relatives or friends	30	14	21	50	36	44
Sound Truck	4	17	12	0	0	0
Film	0	1	1	1	0	0
Pamphlets	0	1	1	1	0	0
Social Worker	1	2	2	28	22	25
Interviewer	5	3	4	1	0	1
Number of Cases	(82)	(117)	(199)	(149)	(123)	(272)

NOTE: Replies were spontaneous and total more than 100 because of multiple responses.

the large increase in new patients apparent from the clinic records is now reconciled—most of the new clinic cases were from other than the four core barrios. On the other hand, there is no difference in place of residence between the ninety-four new cases and the fifty-nine old cases who returned during this period, suggesting that the additional media used in the four core barrios of Las Crucitas did not add much to the radio.

In terms of number of living children, the new clinic cases were very similar to the general population of women of reproductive age. This is both desirable and surprising, since clinics often tend to draw disproportionately from among higher parity women. Since data are lacking on the characteristics of new patients prior to the campaign, whether or not the campaign brought out a lower parity woman than normally attends cannot be determined. But the fact that as many as 43 percent of the new first admissions had only two children or fewer suggests that this might be the case. Further, one-third of the first admissions wanted more children, about the same proportion as in the community prior to the campaign.

As compared with ever-mated women in the barrio census, the new first admissions drew more heavily from women aged 15 — 25 years: 33 percent of the barrio generally, but 46 percent of the new patients. The new admissions may, however, have been somewhat better off economically—55 percent lived in an unattached dwelling unit as opposed to only 32 percent in the census. (This may partly be a reflection of the high proportion coming from outside the core area of Las Crucitas.)

Finally, only one-fourth of the new admissions had practiced birth control before, and one-fifth had attended a family planning clinic elsewhere. In short, *the campaign was essentially drawing new users rather than women seeking a different method.*

Actually, the prospects for use of family planning seem reasonably good. After the campaign one-fourth of the women were currently practicing birth control, most of them by effective methods. Those not using birth control were asked if they plan to use it in the future. Fifty-six percent said "yes." Of these, one-fourth were pregnant and another 10 percent were sterile or wanted more children. A general inclination toward family planning is evident, even if the angle of inclination is not acute.

Conclusions
The provision of family planning facilities in Las Crucitas Health Center was a major step in Honduras' efforts to deal with its popula-

tion problem, important both as a tangible symbol of the government's willingness to come to grips with the problem and as a specific means of reducing the high rate of fertility. Unfortunately, however, the provision of services carries no guarantee that the services will be used, and the six weekly new admissions typical of the clinic in the first half of the year demonstrate that, even when facilities are within walking distance, the community may not be aware of them or care to use them.

The researchers' approach to this problem was twofold: first, to see to what extent an informational campaign could influence the demand for family planning services; and second, to study the characteristics of the community potentially served by the clinic and investigate the general context of health services in Las Crucitas. Over a five-week period in mid-1968, the campaign utilized radio spots for announcements about the family planning clinic, a sound truck with a nurse to answer questions, pamphlet materials, and group meetings. The more general research involved a community census, various sample surveys, and participant observation in the Health Center and the community. In each case there are conclusions which should be relevant for social and health planning.

Conclusions from the Communications Campaign

1. *Short-run, intensive family planning campaigns are feasible in a Latin American setting.* After more than a month of intense utilization of mass media, no public manifestation of disapproval was apparent from individuals or institutions, and the women exposed to the program reacted favorably to this kind of utilization of the mass media.

2. *Short-run, intensive family planning campaigns are relatively economical.* While the total research project, exclusive of the salaries of the two principal investigators, cost $30,000, direct costs for the radio, sound trucks, pamphlets, and film campaign were only $3,000.

3. *Short-run, intensive family planning campaigns can be effective, even among poorly educated slum dwellers.* Weekly attendance at Las Crucitas more than tripled at the height of the campaign, and knowledge of the clinic and attitudes toward family size were intensified or activated.

4. Relative to the other methods employed, and in terms of sheer number of clinic admissions, *radio appears to be the most effective*

agent. This is because of the large number of cases it reached, both within and outside of the study area. The role of the other media is less clear. Other media were less frequently explicitly cited than radio as the source of information on the clinic. On the other hand, the increase in the Las Crucitas clinic case load was much more substantial than at San Felipe, whose clientele were exposed to radio only, rather than sound trucks, pamphlets, etc.

5. *Younger women are ideal targets for family planning information via the mass media.* On the one hand, they normally attend family planning clinics less frequently than do older, higher parity women; and on the other, they seem more responsive and attentive to mass media message than do older women. While it would appear that substantial results can be achieved with relatively little cost and effort, an important qualification should be noted. *It is possible to increase markedly a given clinic's attendance without substantially raising the proportion of the community utilizing its services.* By the end of a campaign, which more than tripled admissions, the fact remained that only 8 percent of the women had ever attended the clinic. In all probability a campaign attracts the better motivated women who need only a slight push to get them moving. In order to attract the "hard-core majority," additional and more long-range kinds of changes may be required. Some of these were apparent from the general study of the community and its health services.

Conclusions from the Community Study

1. *Organizational deficiencies in the clinic can be especially discouraging to patients with low initiative for family planning.* Lack of privacy, excessively informal treatment by staff, and long appointment delays are all guaranteed to discourage potential clientele from visiting the clinic or from returning after the first visit. Such problems most frequently stem from inadequate space and personnel, but even small administrative efficiencies, such as improving the record or appointment system, can accomplish a great deal without great cost.

2. *The heterogeneity of the Las Crucitas population requires a multi-faceted approach to community educational efforts.* At least four important and often overlooked groups in the community were identified who need approaches different from those directed to the "typical" lower class woman of reproductive age.

    a) The transient population. *A good proportion of the barrio population, and this is probably true for most major Latin American cities, should be treated as if they had just arrived and will soon leave.* (One out of every five persons interviewed in the study had arrived within the previous half year, and many moved out between the first and second interviews.) Continuing education and specialized programs are necessary to ensure contacting and influencing such families.

b) Males. As the principal decision makers in the family, male approval is usually required for family planning. *Special programs for males, including the use of male social workers or community organizers, are much needed.*

c) Women without mates. While the typical target of family planning efforts is the married or consensually-mated woman, one-half of the women aged 15 - 44 years were not living in a marital union, although one-half of these were previously doing so. *The potential fertility of the unmarried woman of reproductive age is both a social and demographic problem that cannot be overlooked.*

d) "Educated" residents. A sizable minority (13 percent of household heads) had completed primary school in the barrio, and a number of families had achieved a surprising level of income. Such families not only need to be approached differently as regards family planning information, but *the collaboration of educated residents in community education efforts should be enlisted.*

3. Just as the family planning clinic profits in some ways from the generally good reputation of the Health Center, it also suffers from an image of the Center as being remedial rather than preventive and as being more a place for children's ills than for those of adults. *Both the Health Center and the clinic would profit from community education that stresses the clinic as a place where both children and adults are not only treated for their current ills, but helped to avoid ill health in the future.*

4. *Family planning programs will profit from any successful efforts to mobilize the community in its own behalf on a wide variety of issues.* At the present time, the social isolation and mutual suspicion of many of the barrio's inhabitants, the absence of local leadership, and the pessimism about official efforts to provide adequate water and sanitation facilities all militate against the success of *any* communication effort.

Chapter IV

Honduras Revisited: The Clinic and Its Clientele

Axel I. Mundigo

International Population Program,
Cornell University

In mid-1970 a research team from the International Population Program revisited Honduras and evaluated certain aspects of the government's Maternal and Child Health Program (MCH).* Between the 1968 and 1970 visits, the Honduran family planning program had been strengthened by considerable national and foreign financial support; and its activities had been administratively blended with those of the Department of Maternal and Child Health of the Ministry of Health. An agreement between the MCH Program and the private family planning association (Honduran Family Planning Association) placed responsibility for education and information programs on the latter, but in fact neither group utilized the mass media to any extent.

The MCH Program now operates in public health centers in the nation's larger towns and cities. In addition to family planning, it provides pre-maternal and post-natal services to women and attends children under five years of age. To investigate more fully the functioning of family planning services within this framework, four clinics in Tegucigalpa were selected for three small studies: 1) an analysis of the case cards of a sample of women enrolled in the clinics; 2) a follow-up study of a sample of women who had dropped out of one of these clinics; and 3) a time and motion study of clinic activities.

---

* Based on Chapter VI of "Family Planning in Honduras" by Axel I. Mundigo and J. Mayone Stycos, a report submitted to the U.S. Agency for International Development's Mission to the Republic of Honduras (Contract AID-522-T-211).

Clinic Clientele

To find out who was attending family planning clinics and who was dropping out of them, an analysis was made of the first 800 women enrolling for the first time at four Tegucigalpa clinics in January and February 1970. Of the 800 women who started use of contraception, 40 percent had dropped out after six months. For the purpose of this analysis, drop-out cases are defined as those patients who had failed to come to their respective clinics for their scheduled appointments by mid-August of 1970. In the case of the oral contraceptors, drop-out refers to patients missing at least one (the last) or more of a maximum of three possible appointments. For IUD users, a drop-out case is a woman missing her last appointment, which in most cases was the first after insertion. IUD patients are expected to return to their clinics one month after insertion and then six months later; oral contraceptors return every three months for resupply of pills.

At least two out of every five of the 800 women had used a means of contraception before going to the clinics. In general their tendency was to select the same contraceptive methods they used before entering the Program. Previous IUD users had a greater tendency to drop out than did previous users of other methods; and former IUD users also had a greater tendency to switch to pills (about one-third did so). More of those who had remained active in the Program (48 percent) had been previous users of contraceptives than those who had dropped out (38 percent).

Differences by age and education, as shown in Table IV-1, tend to be negligible when comparing active Program users and drop-outs. The proportion of younger pill drop-outs is only a few

Table IV-1. Age and Education of New Clinic Users,
by Contraceptive Activity

| | Active Users | Drop-outs | | |
		Total	Pill	IUD
Percent under 30 years of age	62	65	68	57
Percent with 3 or more years of education	55	51	50	54
Number of cases	(501)	(299)	(233)	(66)

Source: First 800 new family planning patients at four Tegucigalpa clinics in January and February 1970.

points higher than that of the other groups, and active users were slightly more educated than drop-outs.

Breaking down educational background by type of contraceptive activity (Table IV-2) indicates that for actives and drop-outs in each educational category there is a systematic increase in the proportions below age 30, regardless of activity. This increase is smallest among IUD drop-outs and largest among active users, who reach 98 percent in the most educated group. Among the unschooled these differentials disappear. Since there was no important age difference between active and drop-out groups, other factors must operate that explain this trend. First the younger women had a greater exposure to education than the older women; and secondly, the better education of the younger women gave them a greater awareness of the advantages of planning their families. Table IV-3 clearly supports this. Among the least educated women, the reason given for using contraceptives was to end reproduction—"no more children." Among the more educated the concept of "planning" seemed more clearly defined, and the preference was to "space" children.

Fertility was next examined to ascertain whether the influence of education would produce patterns that might be similar to those observed by age or reason to contracept. Table IV-4 shows, as expected, that fertility declines with increasing levels of education. The average number of pregnancies and of living children was nearly double for women with no schooling as compared to those women

Table IV-2. Women under 30 Years of Age, by Education and Contraceptive Activity

	No Schooling	Primary		More than Primary
		1-2 years	3-6 years	
Percent under 30 years				
Active	50	54	70	98
Dropout				
Pill	48	67	76	82
IUD	48	60	60	63
Number in bases (all ages)				
Active	(117)	(106)	(239)	(39)
Dropout				
Pill	(56)	(60)	(89)	(28)
IUD	(21)	(5)	(23)	(8)

with more than primary education. When comparing women who were active contraceptors with drop-outs, for each educational category except "more than primary," the active women show slightly higher numbers of pregnancies, but some of these differences disappear when comparing the average numbers of living children.

For women with no education the difference between pregnancies and number of living children is about .8 pregnancy; this difference is substantially less among the more educated women whose fertility level was also much lower. In short, the less educated women not only seem to have had a higher fertility level when they

Table IV-3. Reason to Contracept, by Education and Contraceptive Activity (in percent)

Reason	No Schooling		Primary				More than Primary	
			1-2 years		3-6 years			
	A	D	A	D	A	D	A	D
No more children	77	79	69	67	59	62	33	49
Spacing	16	16	27	30	40	35	64	48
Don't know; no answer	7	5	4	3	1	3	3	3
Total	100	100	100	100	100	100	100	100
Number of cases	(117)	(79)	(106)	(66)	(239)	(117)	(39)	(37)
Percent of total cases in each activity category	23	26	21	22	48	39	8	12

NOTE: A= active patients; D= drop-outs.

Table IV-4. Average Number of Pregnancies and Living Children, by Education and Contraceptive Activity

	No Schooling		Primary				More than Primary	
			1-2 years		3-6 years			
	A	D	A	D	A	D	A	D
Average number of pregnancies	5.5	5.3	4.9	4.6	4.1	3.9	2.6	2.9
Average number of living children	4.6	4.6	4.2	4.0	3.5	3.3	2.5	2.5
Number of cases	(117)	(79)	(106)	(66)	(239)	(117)	(39)	(37)

NOTE: A= active patients; D = drop-outs.

went into the Program (or left it) but also seem to have lost a greater part of their reproductive effort.

The small fertility differences between active contraceptors and drop-outs lead to the conclusion that even in reproductive performance, the most important variable with regard to family planning behavior, both groups of women are remarkably similar.

An examination was also made of any differences in patient's characteristics by clinic and any differences among clinics themselves in the services they give. The clinics studied were Alonso Suazo, Las Crucitas, El Manchen, and Villa Adela.

Only small differences existed in the educational level among the clients of the four clinics. About one-half of the women in each clinic (Table IV-5) had three or fewer years of education.

Age and fertility varied little by clinic. The highest mean age was at El Manchen—29 years; and the fertility level of El Manchen users was also highest. Villa Adela serves the least educated population of the four clinics, but its clients seemed to have slightly better child survival rates—60 percent of their pregnancies survived as living children. The only important variation is in the proportions who wanted to space their children; about one-third of the patients at

Table IV-5.   Age, Education, Fertility, and Family Planning, by Clinic

| | Clinic | | | |
	Alonso Suazo	Las Crucitas	El Manchen	Villa Adela
Mean age of patients	28	27	29	27
Percent with 0-3 years education	47	48	39	52
Average number of pregnancies per woman	4.7	4.4	4.9	4.4
Average number of living children per woman	3.6	3.6	4.0	3.7
Percent of women for whom number of pregnancies equals number of living children	52	49	46	60
Average number of infant deaths per woman	.5	.6	.5	.5
Average number of foetal losses per woman	.5	.4	.5	.4
Percent who desire to space children	35	30	2	3
Percent dropping out	44	39	32	19
Percent given IUD	10	11	8	27
Percent receiving Pap test	62	59	34	73
Number of cases	(195)	(340)	(190)	(75)

both Alonso Suazo and Las Crucitas desired to do so, but almost none of those at El Manchen or Villa Adela wanted to space their children.

Having failed to discover important background characteristics among the patients at the four clinics, an examination was made of those indicators that would reflect the quality of the services given by each clinic.

Included with the services, family planning clients at the MCH Program receive a physical examination, a Pap smear test for cancer of the cervix, and a contraceptive fitting or prescription. To carry out the Pap test, the Program has invested in a special cytology laboratory. In a cost-analysis of each service provided by the MCH Program, the Pap test emerged as the single most expensive item. Coincidentally, it is widely believed among lower class populations that the IUD, the most mistrusted contraceptive, produces cancer. In the special survey of Las Crucitas clinic drop-outs, among those who feared a method, 67 percent mentioned the IUD as their most feared contraceptive. (See next section on follow-up activities.) It then seems that clinics showing higher proportions of IUD acceptors are doing a better job in communicating with their patients and possibly eliminating such fears. Table IV-5 shows that not only did the Villa Adela clinic have the highest proportion of women receiving an IUD but also the highest proportion of Pap tests. Villa Adela was also the most successful clinic in keeping its patients active in the Program.

If the success of a family planning clinic is to be measured by the proportions of patients continuing to use its services, Villa Adela stands out as the most and Alonso Suazo as the least successful. To gain more insight into the reasons for the high drop-out rates being experienced by at least three of the four clinics studied, lengthy interviews were conducted with a group of drop-out patients of Las Crucitas clinic. Of the four clinics, Las Crucitas had the largest number of new patients in the period studied; it was not, however, an extreme example of any of the services studied. In sum, while the clientele of these clinics was remarkably similar, the performance of the clinics in retaining them was not.

A Follow-up of Drop-outs from Las Crucitas

At Las Crucitas clinic 85 women were interviewed from a list of 158 MCH Program family planning users who had not returned for their appointments by August of 1970. Some of these women were due to return in June, some in July and some in August. The purpose of the survey was to determine whether social workers (a high-cost resource) could affect return rates. If the survey disclosed that follow-up activities conducted by social workers did not have excellent results in returning women to the MCH Program, then a less expensive resource—auxiliary nurses—should carry out the follow-up work. The survey also sought to disclose the reasons for client drop-out.

Slightly more than one-half of the original list of 158 was interviewed. The proportion of cases who could not be found, 26 percent, is an indicator of the need to improve certain aspects of the intake interview, which occurs when a new patient enters the Program. The address given is often not enough to locate women in neighborhoods such as Las Crucitas. Streets are not marked or even named, and numbers are lacking on most houses. (A good solution is to write down the color or description of the house or the name of another person who will always know the whereabouts of the patient.)

The follow-up survey was carried out between August 29 and September 4, 1970. The interviewers were eight trained social workers and educational personnel of the MCH Program. Of the eighty-five women interviewed, seventeen (20 percent) returned to the clinic to continue treatment in the first twenty days following the end of the interviewing period, and an additional ten (12 percent) came back between the twentieth and fortieth days following the original interview. In all only one-third returned after the follow-up interview. This rate of return is of itself an indicator of the difficulties inherent in returning women who have discontinued use.

One-third of the interviews were done by three male interviewers and the other two-thirds by five female interviewers. Table IV-6 shows that the male interviewers were somewhat more successful in bringing women back to the clinic, both after the twentieth and after the fortieth day.

The average woman drop-out was between 26 and 27 years of age, had four living children, had lost one child in infancy, and had experienced one foetal loss. Two-thirds did not want any more children; among those who wanted more, the majority wanted to space and have only one more. About one-half of the women worked, mostly in the main market selling produce, as servants, or in semi-skilled jobs. Very few were factory workers. Two-thirds knew how to read. One-fourth had never gone to school. About one-half had completed primary school, but only 15 percent had gone be-

Table IV-6.   Drop-out Women Interviewed and Return
              Success, by Sex of Interviewer

	Male Interviewer	Female Interviewer	Total
Percent of women interviewed	33	67	100
Percent returning after 20 days	25	17	20
Percent returning after 40 days	18	9	12
Percent who did not return	57	74	68
Total	100	100	100
Number of cases	(28)	(57)	(85)

yond this level. The proportion who never attended school is slightly larger among those who returned to the clinic than those who did not return.

The husbands were mostly artisans, service personnel or unskilled factory workers. Most of the women were not legally married, and over one-third had more than one marital union. The overall picture is one of a lower class, poorly educated, low income group with a substandard level of living.

The reasons why these MCH Program clients did not return to the clinic should be examined. While 90 percent of the women were primarily pill users, about one-third expressed a desire to switch to another method—usually the IUD or injection. One-third of the prospective switchers felt that the IUD is better than pills; nearly one-half of them declared that the oral contraceptives did not agree with them. Of the total eighty-five women, only 8 percent were pregnant despite the fact that they had stopped going to the clinic. Four of the six IUD patients still had the device in place, and nine of the pill users were obtaining them elsewhere.

None of the women whose husbands had opposed contraceptive use nor any who had work problems returned to the clinic within forty days of the interview (Table IV-7). A majority of those pregnant, of those who mentioned side effects or fear of the contraceptive, and of those whose husbands had left them failed to return. On the other hand, all of those who had forgotten appointments came back. Among those who were still using a method, about one-half returned. When probed specifically on husbands' position with regard to use of contraception, 60 percent of the women declared they had their husbands' permission, 20 percent declared

Table IV-7.   Main Reasons for Not Returning to Clinic
among Selected Drop-out Women (in percent)

	Drop-out Women	Returning Women[a]
Pregnant	11	33
Side effects or fear of method	25	30
Sickness	13	50
Husband left her	10	25
Husband opposes	4	—
Work problems	6	—
Forgot appointment	4	100
Other[b]	22	45
Unknown	5	—
Total	100	
Number of cases	(85)	

Source: Women actually located and interviewed during follow-up survey at Las Crucitas.

[a]   Percent of women in each category returning within 40 days following interview.

[b]   This category includes nine pill users going elsewhere for supplies, six women who still had supplies or were using other methods, and four persons still using an IUD.

their husbands were opposed, and the remainder were uncertain.

In about 50 percent of the drop-out cases interviewed, discontinuation had occurred after the first control visit; and among pill patients 60 percent had stopped contraception six months after beginning use. All of the women interviewed were asked if they had suffered any of a series of specific side effects. As a check on veracity, a presumably fictitious side effect was included—loss of memory. Reassuringly, only three women claimed that side effect. Table IV-8 shows that the least often acknowledged side effect was spotting while the most popular complaint was dizziness. The latter was especially high among returning women, as was complaint of menstrual problems. (It must be noted that returning women were interviewed at the same time as the others, and that the purpose in separating returns from no returns is based on an *a priori* decision to investigate possible differentials in either motivation, or medical, personal, or other reasons to stop going to the clinic.)

Table IV-8.   Side Effects Attributed to
Contraceptive Use (in percent)

Side Effect	Total Sample	Returning Women	Non-returning Women
Spotting	13	15	12
Bleeding	17	19	16
Menstrual problems	32	48	25
Lack of appetite	25	33	21
Dizziness	40	59	32
Nausea	31	41	26
Nervousness	26	26	26
Pains	30	33	28
Number of cases in base	(85)	(27)	(58)

The women were asked if they had heard anything about the method they were using that had prevented them from continuing its use. One-third answered affirmatively. About two-thirds of these said they heard it produces cancer. On the other hand, when asked whether they wanted to continue contraceptive treatment, 90 percent answered affirmatively. Most women were quite ambivalent in their reactions to both oral contraceptives and the IUD. Conflicting information makes it difficult for them to judge, and when in doubt, many discontinue use. The following quotes from the interviewed women illustrate some of these points:

I heard that they produce cancer and hemorrhages but I never had anything. (pill user)

The face gets all spotty. In addition you get cancer and it destroys your nervous system. (pill user)

The IUD produces hemorrhages and it repels the male. It destroys the person's craving. (IUD user)

Among the few women who did not express any desire to return for continued treatment, the reasons were either pregnancy, no husband, or fear of contraceptive side effects. Yet despite an expressed desire to return and a special visit to encourage continued treatment, only one-third of those interviewed had returned to the clinic within forty days following the interview.

Clinic Activity Flow at Las Crucitas and Alonso Suazo

During a four-day period at the Las Crucitas and Alonso Suazo clinics, a time-motion survey was conducted of all patients entering these health centers. Tracer cards were given to each person entering the center. At each major area (reception, doctor, etc.), special personnel filled in the cards with the times of patients' entering or leaving that area. The cards were collected at exit points. More detailed measurements were done within the doctor's office. The accompanying activity flow chart (Figure IV-1) illustrates the various steps that family planning patients take while at these health centers.

In both clinics the first day of the survey was a Monday or a Fri-

Figure IV-1. Activity Flow Chart of Family Planning Patients at the Honduras Maternal and Child Health Program

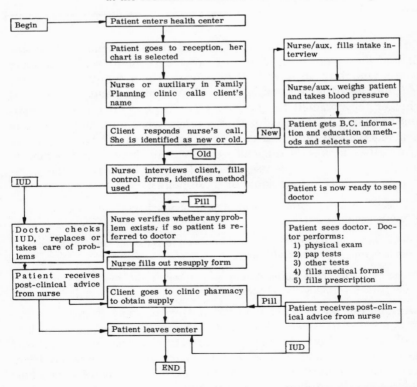

day, the week's busiest days. The second day was a Tuesday or a Wednesday, considered average days. The first day at Las Crucitas (a Friday) registered a total of 436 patients; the second (a Tuesday), 346 patients.In each of these two days, less than 25 family planning patients were served, and the average wait to be seen by a doctor for a new patient was over two and one-half hours. Even for returning contraceptive pill patients who went only to pick up pills, the length of the total visit exceeded two hours.

At Alonso Suazo, 769 persons entered the center the first day (a Monday), and 786 the second day (a Wednesday). These totals exceed by more than 50 percent the estimate given by program officials to the researchers when planning this survey. At Alonso Suazo, as at Las Crucitas, the number of family planning patients served each day was below twenty-five.

The accompanying bar graphs (Figures IV-2, IV-3, and IV-4) illustrate the point that has emerged in the various attempts to locate the sources of the problems facing the MCH Program: most of the

Figure IV-2.   Number of Patients per Day Entering Two Tegucigalpa Health Centers, by Type of Service and Health Center

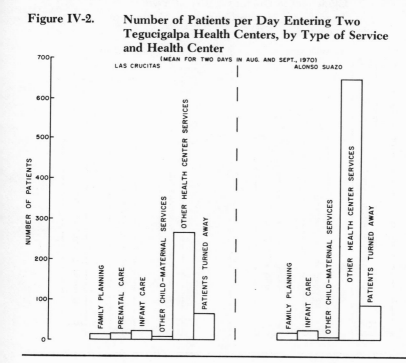

difficulties lie not with the patients but with the clinics. Figure IV-2 reveals that MCH Program patients, as related to total patients coming to the health center, are a small minority—15 percent at Las Crucitas and 6 percent at Alonso Suazo. The need to improve the activity flow at Program clinics is obvious in order to reduce the number of patients who leave unattended.

Figure IV-3 may help to explain why patients leave unattended, why so many drop out of the MCH Program and why new systems must be adopted to improve flow rates. Most patients spend about two hours waiting to see the doctor. The doctor's consultation often takes less than a quarter of an hour. Additional time is spent with nurses, filling out forms, and at the pre-consultation interview and post-talk, but most of a patient's time is spent waiting. A returning pill patient should be expedited by graduate nurses or auxiliaries in minutes instead of the more than two hours her visit usually takes.

Figure IV-3.   **Mean Hours Spent by Family Planning Patients in Clinic and in Doctor's Office at Two Tegucigalpa Health Centers, by Contraceptive Accepted**

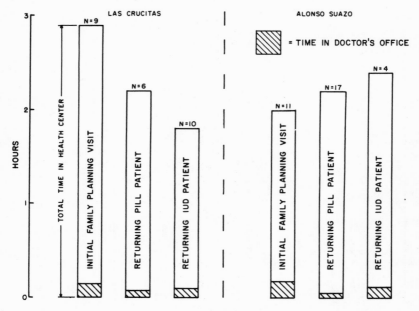

In the survey of follow-up activities at Las Crucitas, it was found that one in five drop-out women were still contracepting. These contraceptors were sufficiently motivated but found it more economical to buy contraceptives than to spend many hours waiting for free pills.

Figure IV-4 is based on selected individual cases rather than on averages or composites. Each bar of the graph shows the distribution of time spent by one patient with the doctor. Nine patients, selected according to types of services the clinic provides, were chosen from Las Crucitas clinic to illustrate the effect of typical and special cases on clinic routines, especially in using up doctor's time in non-medical activities. Each of the doctor's activities at the time these patients were in his office was measured with a stopwatch. Figure IV-4 illustrates one simple fact: from one-third to one-half of the time the doctor spends with the client is spent in form filling. When a case is complicated the examination time remains the same but form filling can take five to six times more than for a regular patient.

Figure IV-4. **Time Spent in Doctor's Office for Nine Selected Patients at Las Crucitas**

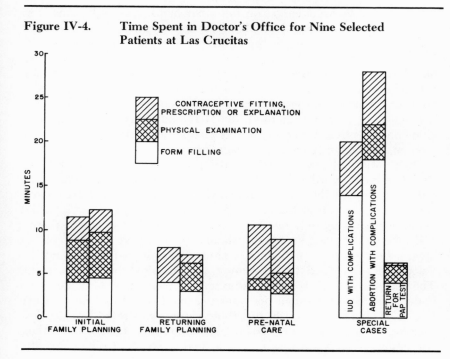

Information and Education

The interviews at Las Crucitas revealed that contraceptive information originated entirely from neighbors and friends. *The clinic at Las Crucitas was not mentioned.* These results underscore the need for a completely revitalized effort by the MCH Program in the area of education. While contraceptives do produce some side effects, no empirical evidence exists to support the exaggerated claims made by some people. The Program's effort in cancer detection should be better publicized so that fear of a supposed cancer-producing device can be eliminated. Then perhaps a woman who is already motivated to use family planning methods will not so readily drop out of the program when she hears erroneous claims from friends and neighbors.

The concept of responsible parenthood has had wide acclaim everywhere because it is also acceptable to Roman Catholics. Among the eighty-four women interviewed from the Las Crucitas clinic the concept had very low saliency; less than one in five had heard about it. Among the few who had heard of responsible parenthood, only one-third really knew its meaning.

Contraceptive knowledge, on the other hand, was high. This is to be expected, however, since all of these women had used at least one method. Knowledge of the contraceptive pill was universal, the IUD was second and, surprisingly, the injection third. At least one-third of the women had heard of the contraceptive injection. While knowledge of contraceptives was high, fear of them was also high. One-half of the women expressed such feelings (Table IV-9). Among those fearing a method, the IUD ranked as the least acceptable contraceptive. While much less anxiety existed among returning women, they nevertheless had misgivings.

Distribution of contraceptives without educating the users is a double-edged sword. The fears expressed are not surprising when only one-third of the women acknowledged having received contraceptive information at the clinic. Even worse, among those who did get an explanation, only one-half understood what was said to them.

Education at the clinic level should be effective at least in the areas where most women show a natural curiosity—the acts and developments that lead to pregnancy and eventual birth of a child. The proportion of women interviewed from Las Crucitas who understood how a woman becomes pregnant was only one in every five. The clinic could easily distribute simply illustrated booklets explaining not only the basic physiological facts and their consequences, but also the means available for controlling fertility.

Only a minority of the women interviewed acknowledged receiving any family planning literature.

The women were asked to give an opinion of the services and personnel at the Las Crucitas clinic. (Because some of the questions were asked by personnel identified with the clinic, the results may present a biased picture.) Nearly 90 percent of the women said that they had been well treated during their last visit to the clinic; little difference was noted in this regard between those who returned and those who did not. However, nearly 90 percent of those who returned and only 80 percent of those who did not return said that they had been well treated by the auxiliary nurse. Similar differences exist for their evaluations of doctor, nurse, and receptionist performance.

When asked whether anything ought to be done to improve the services at the clinic, 40 percent of those who returned answered affirmatively, but only 20 percent of the non-returning women

Table IV-9.   Family Planning Attitudes and Knowledge (in percent)

	Total Sample	Returning Women	Non-returning Women
Prefer pills	44	46	44
Prefer IUD	22	29	19
Express fear of contraceptive methods	52	42	56
Fear pills (among those who fear a method)	19	10	22
Fear IUD (among those who fear a method)	67	80	63
Claimed that they received an explanation of family planning methods at the clinic	33	38	32
Claimed they did not understand what was explained to them (among those who received an explanation)	48	44	50
Claimed to know how a woman becomes pregnant	23	25	23
Gave evidence of knowing how a woman becomes pregnant (among those declaring to know)	21	33	15
Claimed to have received family planning literature during their visits to the clinic	38	29	42
Approximate number of cases	(81)	(57)	(24)

agreed. One-half of the non-returning women who said that improvements were needed indicated that they were unhappy with the quality of service. Some of the returning women suggested improvements in the areas of education and distribution and availability of specific contraceptives. Users complained about changes in brands of oral contraceptives issued by the clinic. Certain brands are distrusted, and users who are content with one type of pill are extremely reluctant to change.

The following are clinic improvements suggested by the interviewed women:

> The clinic ought to offer a variety of contraceptive treatments to be able to select, and better treatment should be given to the users.

> The person who is in charge of dispensing the medicines should take the time to explain how to use them.

> They should install curtains to make it more private.

> There should be more understanding for us humble people because we go there with great fear.

> They should show movies while one waits.

The survey of Las Crucitas drop-outs gives additional evidence that a great part of the reason family planners drop out of the Program is the clinics themselves. Las Crucitas is one of the MCH Program's largest urban clinics. It is in a highly populated, lower class neighborhood. A much greater effort is needed in both clinic organization and outside information and education to successfully reinforce the motivation of family planners, to improve their family planning knowledge and finally to keep them in the Program.

Conclusions

Results from the surveys reported in this chapter reinforce each other in locating the source of the Honduras Maternal and Child Health Program clinic operational problems. The premise that the most important goal of a family planning program is, after attracting patients, keeping them active was used as the yardstick by which clinic performance was measured. The first survey of 800 new family planners at four urban clinics in 1970 showed that 40 percent had dropped out of the service within six months. Age, education, and parity of drop-outs were no different from those who continued to regularly attend the Program clinics. The difference in drop-out rates among clinics (from 19 percent to 44 percent) indicates that a woman's experience in the clinic may have much to do with whether or not she returns. The follow-up survey at Las Crucitas, one of the Program's largest urban clinics, demonstrated the poor performance of the clinic in educating and reaching its clients—only one-third of the patients acknowledged having received proper instructions on the contraceptive method they were using, and 10 percent were obtaining their resupplies elsewhere. Time-motion surveys at two busy Tegucigalpa health centers indicate that while the new patient spends about fifteen minutes in the doctor's office, she spends almost three hours in the center, most of it waiting. A patient returning only for a supply of pills spends over two hours in the center. These delays defy the strongest motivation and point to the need for improving patient stream rates, improving clinic services, and enlarging the scope of information and education programs.

Chapter V

Information Campaigns and the Growth of Family Planning in Colombia

Alan B. Simmons

Department of Sociology,
York University, Toronto

Colombia is widely regarded as one of the most traditional of the larger nations in Latin America. Nineteenth-century parties (the Liberals and the Conservatives) still dominate the political system; the Roman Catholic Church is strong; and the landowning and propertied families have held their power in the face of populist movements and widespread internal violence. Nevertheless, since 1965 two family planing programs—one private and the other part of the government-sponsored maternal health program—have developed rapidly in Colombia and now provide a web of services throughout the nation. Both programs are using or planning public information services to support their clinics. A conservative national context, the existence of large scale family planning services, and mass media experimentation all make Colombia a valuable setting for evaluating new clinics and the role that various communication techniques may have in attracting new patients.

An Overview of Family Planning Programs in Colombia

Policy and Organization since 1965[1]

The origins of family planning programs in Colombia may be traced in great part to the activities of a small corps of medical doctors living in the principal cities of the nation. Prior to 1965 only a few economic planners had noted the dangers of Colombia's rapid rate of population growth, a rate in excess of 3 percent annually in recent years.[2] In 1965 a group of physicians, under the energetic leadership of Dr. Fernando Tamayo, set up the Association for the Welfare of the Colombian Family (PROFAMILIA) affiliated with the International Planned Parenthood Federation and opened a pilot clinic (Centro Piloto) in Bogota. By 1970, PROFAMILIA had twenty-four clinics[3] in major urban areas throughout the country, which were inscribing new patients at a rate of about 4,000 per month.

Also in 1965 the Colombian Association of Medical Schools (ASCOFAME) established a division of population studies. Founded in 1959 by the medical schools of the nation, ASCOFAME was created to improve university medical research and education by modifying the teaching emphasis on individual medical practice and by introducing a new emphasis on social medicine and maternal health problems. A new focus on population change—migration, mortality, and fertility—complemented ASCOFAME's general interest in social medicine. Although it is an independent professional organization, ASCOFAME's family planning activities became closely associated with government policies and programs; hence the evolution of both activities may be discussed together.

Under the dynamic leadership of Hernan Mendoza, ASCOFAME's Division of Population Studies initiated a program of research on abortion, fertility, and the practice of birth control. The division also translated into Spanish a large number of foreign books and papers dealing with population problems and family planning.[4] The research indicated high levels of induced abortions and showed that women generally wanted smaller families and were interested in family planning.[5] The translations often dealt with the dangers of rapid population growth and argued that training in family planning should be an essential part of a physician's education. ASCOFAME also hosted two conferences—the first Pan-American Assembly of Population (Cali, August 1965) and the First International Conference on Family Planning (Popayan, September 1966)—where foreign and national experts discussed population problems and ways to attack them. Finally, ASCOFAME presented the Ministry of Health with a proposal for the training of medical personnel and for initiating several pilot family planning centers for research and training. The Ministry accepted the proposal, and in September 1966, signed a contract with the Pan-American Health Organization and ASCOFAME to have it carried out. Thus, the government began to support family planning without having to confront its critics in seeking an official policy on the matter. Colombian President Lleras Restrepo publicly pointed out that ASCOFAME was an independent organization whose policies he could not control; he thus was able to advise the Roman Catholic

Church to convey its criticism of "artificial" methods of birth control directly to ASCOFAME[6].

In June 1967, the Ministry of Health authorized ASCOFAME to train personnel and develop programs of maternal health, including family planning, in the nation's 340 public health centers. The development of an organization for family planning services within the health centers is still underway. By the spring of 1970 about one-half of the clinics were issuing regular reports on their family planning activities, indicating that some services were being provided in at least the regions served by these clinics. By effectively handling opposition in the early stages of the program, the government has been willing to take increasing responsibility for it. As a final step in the expansion of family planning facilities, in 1968 ASCOFAME began organizing and training maternal hospital personnel for post-partum family planning education and service programs. Twenty-one hospitals in major urban centers were participating in this program by the spring of 1970. In April 1969, the Ministry of Health officially declared family planning to be part of maternal health services in the 340 health care areas throughout the nation.

It is difficult to evaluate the progress of clinics in the ASCOFAME-government program, for most of the data relating to the progress of these clinics are confidential. However, preliminary data indicate wide variations among clinics in the number of new patients—a range of from one or two per month to 150 or more. The total monthly inflow for all 340 clinics was probably no more than 5,000 in early 1970, in contrast to 4,000 per month for PROFAMILIA. The government post-partum program may account for an additional 3,000 per month.[7] Based on these crude estimates it would appear that the PROFAMILIA program with twenty-four clinics currently accounts for about one-third of the total new patients, the 340 government clinics account for another 40 percent, and the 21 government post-partum programs account for the remainder. It is of interest that the PROFAMILIA Centro Piloto clinic in Bogota alone has handled up to 1,600 new patients per month in peak periods. In other words three or four clinics of the size and location of Centro Piloto could handle as many patients as all 340 government clinics were accepting in 1970.

The Expansion of the PROFAMILIA Clinic System

Beginning in 1965 with the Centro Piloto in Bogota, the PROFAMILIA clinic system expanded slowly at first. By the beginning of 1968 a second clinic, Hospital San José, had been added in Bogota, and two others had been established in Medellin and Barranquilla. Since early 1968, clinic expansion has been rapid, and by the end of 1969 there were twenty-four clinics in seventeen cities. The growth of new patients in this period has been correspondingly rapid. While about 18,000 new patients entered the PROFAMILIA clinics in 1968, nearly 42,000 new patients entered in 1969 (Figure V-1).

Centro Piloto, the first and still the largest clinic, grew very quickly over the first year and a half. By the first quarter of 1967 it was accepting more than 1,600 new patients each month, but over the next two years the number of new patients declined steadily. In the last quarter of 1968 only one-half as many new patients entered as during the peak inflow in the first quarter of 1967, nearly two years previously. During 1969 the number of patients again increased, almost to 1967 levels. Since the third quarter of 1969 the number of new patients has again fallen off. The sudden rise in new patients and the subsequent decline over the year 1969 is particularly noteworthy because the period of rapid growth corresponds closely to

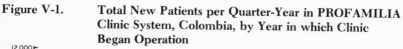

Figure V-1. Total New Patients per Quarter-Year in PROFAMILIA Clinic System, Colombia, by Year in which Clinic Began Operation

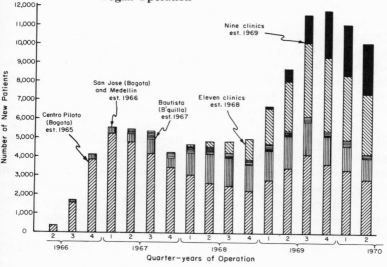

the period in which the services of the Centro Piloto were announced twenty times daily on as many as five radio stations in Bogota.

In 1966 PROFAMILIA established a clinic in Medellin and a second clinic in Bogota (Hospital San José). Despite the different settings these two clinics showed rapid growth in the first two quarters, subsequently evidencing rapid declines to negative growth rates in excess of 30 percent by the fifth quarter of operation (Figure V-1). More recently, these clinics have shown some fluctuation at low positive and negative growth rates. The Medellin clinic seems to have stabilized at roughly 333 new patients per month and San José seems to have stabilized at around 175.

In 1967 only the Bautista clinic in Barranquilla was added. Although located in a city of 700,000, the Bautista clinic has never attracted large numbers of patients. In the second quarter of operation it accepted a high of nearly 400 patients, but since then the number has declined and appears to have stabilized at around 250 to 300 new patients per quarter. Whether this low intake is due to the characteristics of the clinic or to the distinctive Caribbean culture along the coastal region (predominately Negro and Mulatto population with high rates of consensual unions and illegitimacy) is not known.

Eleven new clinics were established in 1968. Among them an additional clinic (Atlantico) was established at Barranquilla and a third clinic was opened in Bogota. The others were opened in various intermediate or large cities around the nation: Armero, Cucuta, Ibague, Neiva, Pasto, Sogamoso, Puerto Berrio, Buenaventura, and Bucaramanga. These clinics have shown considerable variation in growth patterns. Some have grown rapidly and, as the new clinic in Barranquilla, appear still to be in a growth phase. Others have grown less rapidly but have continued to expand (Armero, for example). Most, however, have shown moderately rapid growth in the first three quarters of operation and then large actual declines in new patients arriving in the third quarter of 1969. Since many of these communities had their clinic facilities announced by radio in 1969, possibly the initiation and termination of the radio campaign help explain these swings in case load. Despite their diverse patterns of growth, clearly the clinics established in 1968 have contributed greatly to the overall PROFAMILIA effort by nearly doubling the number of new patients who were attracted by clinics established in previous years.

In 1969 nine more clinics were added bringing the total number of PROFAMILIA clinics to twenty-four. Five of these new clinics are located in Bogota; and Cali, the only remaining large Colombian city that had been without PROFAMILIA services, opened its first clinic in 1969. The other clinics were opened in several intermediate size cities: Armenia, Manizales, Pereira, and Monteria. While it is difficult to establish firm trends for recently organized clinics, they tend toward rapid growth, and these newer clinics averaged more than 250 new patients each in the most recent quarter. Their overall effect then has been to add more than 2,500 new patients to the PROFAMILIA total in the second quarter of 1969.

In 1969 PROFAMILIA began its post-partum program in the maternity unit of the Social Security Hospital in Bogota. This effort has been remarkably successful, providing family planning services to roughly 600 women per month. However, the manner in which new patients are obtained differs so radically from the conditions under which new patients are obtained in the clinics that the post-partum programs have been excluded from the data in Figure V-1.

The PROFAMILIA program apparently favors the use of the intra-uterine device (IUD).[8] Though there is some variation between clinics, only the clinic in Medellin prescribes oral contraceptives even one-half as often as the IUD; and for all clinics the overall ratio of IUD to pill acceptors is approximately ten to one. The diaphragm appears to be offered only in the Centro Piloto, Bogota, and even there it is provided to less than 2 percent of the new patients. Experiments with injections have begun in several clinics but these account for less than 3 percent of new patients in the most recent period.

To summarize, most of the growth in the number of new patients over the past five years is due to the expansion in number of clinics. The Centro Piloto, which opened in Bogota in 1965, reached its peak number of new patients by early 1967 and has subsequently experienced overall decline. New clinics added in Bogota, Medellin, and Barranquilla, made an important contribution to growth, but the inflow of these clinics taken together never equalled more than one-half of the Centro Piloto inflow. The overall number of new patients did not substantially increase until a total of twenty new clinics were added to the system in 1968 and 1969. While many of these new clinics are small, both because they are new and because many are located in smaller cities or in larger cities where clinics previously existed, the total impact has been no more than to double the number of new patients.

The number of new cases usually increases rapidly for the first few quarters of operation of a new clinic but tends to level off or even decline after a year or two. However, in the most recent calendar year of operation, 1969, extremely rapid growth of new patients was due both to the opening of new clinics and to an increase in new patients in older clinics. The extent to which this surge in case loads can be attributed to mass media campaigns is a question that will be investigated subsequently.

Despite the rapid growth in new patients the proportion of mated fecund women served in the nation as a whole is only about 4 percent. As Table V-1 shows, however, the proportion is much higher in those cities where the PROFAMILIA effort has been concentrated. For example, in Bogota, where roughly 11 percent of the nation's population lives, *close to 20 percent of the mated women aged 15 — 49 years appear to have accepted birth control at PROFAMILIA clinics in the past five years.* An additional 2 percent has accepted the IUD in the PROFAMILIA post-partum program. In the other cities where the clinics are more recently established or

---

Table V-1.   First Admissions in PROFAMILIA
Clinics as a Percent of Mated Women Aged 15-49
in Six Cities and the Nation

Place (and date first clinic was established)	Estimated Population July 1970 [a]	Estimated Number of Mated Women Aged 15-49, July 1970 [b]	Total Number of New Clinic Patients to June 30, 1970 [c]	Percent of New Patients of Mated Women Aged 15-49
Bogota (1965)	2,529,560	315,689	61,496	19.5
Medellin (1966)	1,102,497	137,591	11,402	8.2
Barranquilla (1967)	650,411	81,171	5,663	7.0
Bucaramanga (1968)	319,763	39,906	4,845	12.1
Cucuta (1968)	241,673	30,161	2,918	9.7
Cali (1969)	926,456	115,621	2,906	2.5
Colombia	21,449,000	2,676,835	109,418	4.1

[a]   Estimated from the July 1964 census, projecting growth to June 1970 on the basis of the continuous rate of increase for each place between the census of May 1951 and that of July 1964, where $P_2/P_1 = e^{rn}$.

[b]   Estimate from the proportion of the urban population aged 15-49 reported married or in free unions at the time of the 1964 census.

[c]   This includes clinic patients only. Post-partum patients are excluded.

where there are fewer clinic facilities relative to the population, the impact of the program has been smaller.[9]

The estimates in Table V-1 should be treated cautiously. Not all the patients who accept birth control in a given clinic are from the city where the clinic is located. Bogota is surrounded by several hundred small towns from which some of the patients probably come. Moreover, what has been designated as the eligible population (mated women aged 15 — 49 years) may not well define the population that actually is in need of birth control. On the one hand, many women may be practicing birth control on their own, and, on the other, many women who list themselves as "single" or "separated" may have children and currently be at risk of further pregnancies. While the proportion who go to the PROFAMILIA clinic might be reduced by the availability of government clinics, in the absence of data on these programs, it is impossible to evaluate what their contributions have been. Finally, not all the women who have received help from the PROFAMILIA clinics can be assumed to be still using birth control. The effects of the clinic's activities on actual birth planning and levels of fertility is a subject beyond the scope of the present investigation.

Despite these reservations, it seems fair to conclude that after a few years of operation the longer established PROFAMILIA clinics have reached from 7 to 20 percent of the mated women of fecund age in the communities they serve.

Patterns of Clinic Growth in the Absence of Information Campaigns

To examine the "natural" pattern of clinic growth in the absence of information campaigns specifically designed to attract new patients, growth rates for each quarter-year of operation were calculated for the four oldest clinics. In Figure V-2 the growth rates are shown from time of clinic inception to the beginning of the radio information campaign in the first quarter of 1969. Centro Piloto, because it was established before the others, operated longer before the radio campaign and gives us the best picture of a "natural" growth trend.

Figure V-2 shows that the larger clinics tend to have higher growth rates in the initial period of rapid expansion than do the smaller clinics. Centro Piloto is the largest clinic, Medellin is the second, San José the third, and Bautista is the smallest. Growth rates in the initial first quarters of operation directly reflect these size differences. Secondly, the patterns of growth over time are remarkably similar,

Figure V-2. Growth of New Patients by Quarter-Years of Clinic Operation at Four Principal PROFAMILIA Clinics Prior to the Radio Campaign

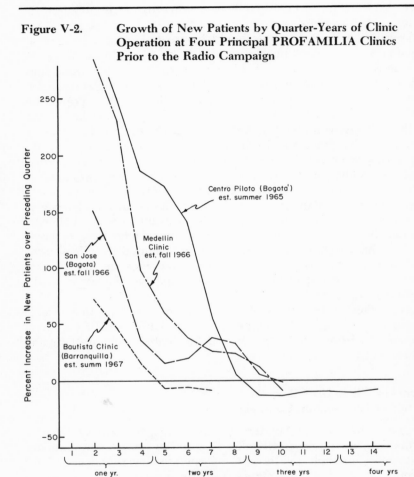

NOTE: Data was smoothed by calculating a moving average over three quarter-years of operation.

at least for the three larger clinics. Growth rates are initially high and then quickly decline; after two or two and one-half years of operation they actually become negative. Prior to the information campaign, Centro Piloto experienced nearly two years of a 10 to 15 percent negative growth rate per quarter. Thus, while the cumulative number of women served by the clinic was still rising, the number added each month was gradually declining. A continued 10 to 15 percent decline per quarter-year is sufficient to reduce the number of new patients arriving by 50 percent in about a year and one-half. While the length of operation of the Medellin and the San José clinics was not long enough prior to the information campaign to see if they too would continue to show negative growth rates, their similarities to the Centro Piloto clinic for the period that they can all be compared suggests that they too would have shown negative rates. The Bautista clinic deviates from the general pattern only in the short period that elapsed between inauguration and the plunge to negative growth rate.

To explore the generality of the investigation's findings, similar growth rates were calculated for five private Mexico City clinics of the Fundación para Estudios de la Población (FEPAC).[10] Since there have been no information campaigns in Mexico, it was possible to chart these rates from the inauguration of each clinic to the second quarter of 1969, the last period for which data were available. These growth rates for each clinic by quarter-year of operation are shown in Figure V-3. La Villa, the oldest and largest clinic in the Mexico City system, does not follow the Colombian pattern very well. Although growth rates began declining for La Villa about a year after it was established, growth rates in the initial period were never really high; but despite a gradual decline they are still positive three years after the clinic began. The pattern for the other clinics, however, comes closer to the Colombian model, and the two most recently established clinics (Moctexuma and Penon) seem to be starting a course that will follow the Colombian pattern rather closely. Both these latter clinics began with very rapid rates of growth that declined steeply within one year to low negative rates of growth.

The preceding analysis strongly suggests that there is a natural tendency for clinic growth to stabilize and even to become negative in a year or two. If there were no limits on the capacity of a clinic to accept new patients and if a diffusion model were in operation (in other words, with greater numbers of women entering and spreading the news to their friends who in turn came for assistance), one would expect continuing high rates of growth. Is the fact that this does not happen attributable to a clinic's limited capacity or to the fact that family planning did not catch on as the diffusion model suggests?

The capacity of the clinic to accept new patients is affected by the requirement that contraceptive acceptors return for periodic checkups, usually at least every six months. With a fixed clinic staff,

Figure V-3.   Growth of New Patients by Quarter-Year of Clinic
               Operation at Five FEPAC Clinics in Mexico City

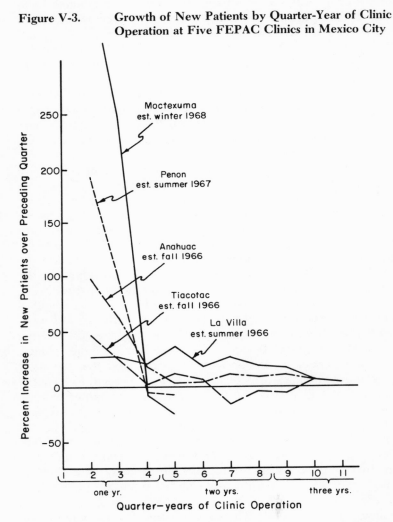

NOTE: Data was smoothed by calculating a moving average over three
quarter-years of operation.

the size of the accumulated active clinic population will influence a
clinic's ability to deal with new patients. When a clinic first begins,
it has no accumulated population for which it must provide checkups; but after several years of operation a very large proportion of

the clinic's time may be spent in this task alone. Thus, in the Cali clinic (established in 1969), by the second quarter of 1970 59 percent of all patients were previous acceptors coming in for checkups. But in the long established Centro Piloto in Bogota, for the same period, old patients accounted for no less than 87 percent of all patients handled! Large numbers of old patients could thus help to account for the decline in the number of new patients because facilities are too limited to accept them.

From descriptive reports on the operation of the PROFAMILIA clinics, it is clear that the older clinics in Colombia are frequently crowded and the women must occasionally wait several hours for an appointment.[11] Moreover, the "routine" cancer cytology (Pap smear) test and vaginal exam may be too much for some women, and the spread of gossip about them may discourage others from going to the clinic. While these negative attitudes may serve to discourage many women from going to a clinic, it is nevertheless apparent that other factors (such as a public information campaign) can greatly increase the number of new patients even in older crowded clinics like Centro Piloto. Thus, the conclusion must be made that facilities in these older clinics are not completely inelastic to increased demand, for when the number of women demanding service increases, somehow the clinics do manage to expand their staff, streamline the procedure, or crowd in the patients. Rapid increases in new patients exemplifying this pattern were noted in Centro Piloto, Medellin, and the Barranquilla-Atlantico clinic in the first two quarters of 1969 shortly after the radio campaign began.

In conclusion it would appear that the natural course of growth in the absence of directed informational campaigns is characterized by a gradual leveling off in the number of new patients and eventual steady declines in these new numbers within any given clinic. While diffusion of information may be taking place naturally through word of mouth, it is apparent that either this process reaches only a few people or that it must be supplemented by other forms of education and persuasion. The data suggest a growth model where, prior to the inauguration of the clinic facilities, a "backlog" of women accumulates waiting for family planning services. When the clinics open and word spreads, these women begin to flow to the clinic in ever increasing numbers. However, within a year the "backlog" of highly motivated women begins to be reduced, and the number of new patients begins to decline. Perhaps the less motivated do not seek information and remain ignorant about the clinic facilities. Alternatively, the information about the clinic may be spread, but the remaining eligible women may be less interested than the first waves. Whatever the reason, of great importance is the means that will bring these less motivated women into the clinic. The two means traditionally utilized by Health Education specialists—pamphlet materials and direct personal visitation—will be examined.

A Pilot Experiment in Family Planning Communications

Although the prime interest in the Colombian setting was radio, the researchers wished to have some rough measure of the comparative effectiveness of other traditional methods of communication. Accordingly, a small experiment was designed to assess the relative impact on clinic attendance of (a) a personal visit by a family planning educator, and (b) the delivery of written materials on family planning. Both were designed to carry much more information on family planning than was feasible in radio programming.

Experimental Design

From a list of lower and middle class Bogota women of known characteristics, 881 were chosen aged 15 − 44 years with at least one child. These women were then assigned at random to one of three groups. 1) *Pamphlets:* The women of this group received three pamphlets about birth control along with a letter and a coupon directing them to the services at the Centro Piloto family planning clinic, all delivered by messenger to their homes. 2) *Visits:* Home visits were paid by a family planning worker who spent an average of ten minutes discussing family planning and encouraging a visit to the clinic. The women were also given the pamphlet materials and coupon. 3) *Control:* The women of this group received no information.[12]

The coupon reminded the women when and where they could obtain family planning service and helped the researchers identify the women who entered the clinic in response to the communication, since they had been asked to bring the coupon with them. However, to identify women in the control group (who received no coupon) as well as women in the experimental groups who forgot to bring the coupon to the clinic, the names and addresses of all women in the study were compared with the names and addresses of all women entering the clinic as new patients in the six-month period after the communication was delivered. Information on the characteristics of the women who entered the clinic in this period was obtained from a basic clinic interview normally conducted for all new clinic patients covering family income, education, husband's age, and prior contraceptive practice.

The experiment was carried out at the Centro Piloto clinic between August 1 and August 30, 1969, under the general supervision of Rigmor Anderson, a Cornell University graduate student. The three workers on the experiment were hired and trained by PROFAMILIA. The two family planning workers had previously worked for a year as interviewers in a national fertility survey and had already obtained a good deal of experience in discussing family planning matters with women.

Table V-2 indicates the size of the final sample in the different social strata and shows the number of women approached in each group and the rate of non-response.[13]

Table V-3 examines several characteristics of the women who were actually contacted including age, number of living children, education, employment, marital status, and economic status. At least for the characteristics examined, no substantial differences between the groups were found, indicating that the random assignment was successful despite differential non-response.

Results of the Experiment

The percentage of women who responded to the study's informational campaign by visiting PROFAMILIA in the six-month period after the information was delivered is given in Table V-4. Several eligibility definitions are used to obtain a more detailed assessment of the effect of the communication. First, the women who almost certainly would not respond—sterile women and those who had already attended a clinic—were removed from the eligible population. Then, moving into less certain factors, women were excluded who claimed they wished to have more children. Next, women who were very young (15—19 years) or old (40+ years), were removed, first to make the results more comparable to similar studies involving women between the ages of 20 and 39, and second because women outside the age range 20 to 39 seem less likely to seek family planning advice. (See the characteristics of women responding to the radio campaign, in the section The Radio Campaign in Colombia.)

The first finding concerns the low response to either communication method. Out of 557 women who received either the pamphlet materials or the family planning worker's visit, only 17 women (about 3 percent) actually went to the Centro Piloto clinic in the six months following the communication. However, just over two-thirds could be categorized as "unlikely" to go to the clinic because they believed themselves infertile, because they had already been to a clinic, because they wanted more children, or because they were using birth control. Eleven percent of the visit group believed that

Table V-2. Sample Design and Non-Response among Women in Pilot Family Planning Communication Study, August 1969, by Economic Status

	Control	Pamphlet	Visit	Total
Number of women sampled				
Middle class	51	42	66	159
Lower middle class	32	48	65	145
Lower class	199	214	164	577
Total	282	304	295	881
Number of non-respondents a				
Middle class	15	11	10	36
Lower middle class	2	2	5	9
Lower class	8	9	5	22
Total	25	22	20	67
Percent non-response				
Middle class	29	26	15	23
Lower middle class	6	4	8	6
Lower class	4	4	3	4
Total	9	7	6	7
Number included in pilot study				
Middle class	36	31	56	123
Lower middle class	30	46	60	136
Lower class	191	205	159	555
Total	257	282	275	814

a Women sampled who could not be contacted for various reasons.

Table V-3. Characteristics of Women in Pilot Study (in percent)

	Control	Pamphlet	Visit	Total
Age				
15-24 years	24	27	25	25
25-34 years	45	48	46	47
35-44 years	31	25	29	28
Total	100	100	100	100
Number of Living Children				
1-2	37	42	41	40
3-4	31	32	26	30
More than 4	32	26	33	30
Total	100	100	100	100
Education				
0-3 years	33	34	33	33
4-6 years	38	45	42	42
7-12 years	29	21	25	25
Total	100	100	100	100
Employment				
Working	25	25	23	25
Not working	75	75	77	75
Total	100	100	100	100
Marital Status				
Married	88	90	86	88
Single, separated, widowed, divorced	12	10	14	12
Total	100	100	100	100
Economic Status				
Middle class	14	11	20	15
Lower middle class	12	16	22	17
Lower class	74	73	58	68
Total	100	100	100	100
Number of cases	(257)	(282)	(275)	(814)

they could not have more children, 19 percent had been to a clinic before the campaign, and another 24 percent were using birth control at the time of the experiment. Thus a high proportion of the sample seems to have been well informed on birth control, probably as a result of the PROFAMILIA services and other educational efforts. Nevertheless, the low response cannot be attributed only to such ineligibility criteria, for, when all of the "unlikely to come" women are removed, the proportion of those remaining who went to the clinic is still only about 7 percent.

Differences between the control group and the experimental groups moreover are very small. With all less eligible women removed, 5 percent of the control group went, while only 7 percent

Table V-4. Acceptance Rates by Treatment and Eligibility Definition for Women in Pilot Study (in percent)

Eligibility Definition	Treatment			
	Control	Pamphlet	Visit	Total
1	2.0	2.8	3.3	2.7
2	2.2	3.2	3.6	3.1
3	2.6[a]	3.7[a]	4.2	3.5
4	2.7[a]	4.0[a]	4.5	3.8
5	2.9[a]	4.3[a]	5.0	4.1
6	3.8	5.0	5.7	4.8
7	5.2[a]	6.6[a]	7.6	6.5
Number of acceptors	5	8	9	22

NOTE: The eligibility definitions are as follows:
1. Total number of currently-mated women 15-44 years with at least one child (N+814).
2. Less 11 percent of total who believe they are unable to have children for medical reasons.
3. Further less 15 percent of women in "2" who attended PROFAMILIA before August 1, 1969.
4. Further less 6 percent of women in "3" who attended another family planning clinic before August 1, 1969.
5. Further less 8 percent of women in "4" who want more children now.
6. Further less 15 percent of women in "5" who were 19 years of age and younger or 40 years and older.
7. Further less 45 percent of women in "6" who were using a birth control method, but were not going to a clinic.
[a] Denominator estimated from the distribution of the visit group.

of the pamphlet and 8 percent of the visit group responded (Table V-4). While these differences are in the expected direction, they are not statistically significant at the .05 level, and substantively they are of no consequence. In other words, the information campaign did not significantly alter the rate of acceptance that could have been expected in the absence of an information campaign.

Characteristics of Women Responding

Table V-5 shows small but consistent differences between the general population and women who normally go to the clinic. Women who first attended the clinic in July and August of 1969 were somewhat younger, less educated, less likely to be working, of somewhat higher parity, and less likely to want more children than average women in Bogota; and those from the experimental group who responded to the information campaign fall between the normal clinic population and the average women in Bogota on these characteristics. However, the women from the experimental groups showed higher parity, in the three- to four-children range, and were clearly less likely to desire more children. These findings suggest that de-

Table V-5. Selected Characteristics of Women in Pilot Study, Women Who Responded to Information Campaign, and All New Clinic Patients for July and August 1969 (in percent)

	Women in Experimental Groups (Control, Pamphlets, Visit)	Women Who Attended Clinic in Response to Pamphlet or Visit	All New Clinic Patients for July-August 1969
Under 30 years of age	47	54	62
Less than four years of school	34	40	41
Working	25	19	10
Want more children	16	4	10
Number of living children			
1-2	40	35	31
3-4	29	46	36
5+	31	19	33
Number of cases	(814)	(26)[a]	(1,124)

[a] This includes seventeen cases from the pamphlet and visit groups plus an additional nine cases who responded to a separate pilot information campaign involving pamphlets only.

spite the low response to the information campaign, the few women who did respond more closely reflect the characteristics of the female population of Bogota than does the overall clinic population. It may well be that normal channels of communication are less effective in reaching older, better educated, lower parity women. More likely, these women are less likely to require help. These hypotheses will be further explored in the next section.

Conclusions

It may be helpful to contrast these data with the results of other similar communication experiments. Two previous studies seem particularly useful for this purpose. The first is the Taichung experiment carried out in Taichung, Taiwan, in 1963[14] and involved various media (posters, group meetings, home visits, and pamphlets), focused on an entire community, lasted nine months, and was intensely concentrated. Nine family planning clinics were involved. The experiment revealed a somewhat higher response rate than did the Colombian study—7 percent for the control group, 7 percent for the pamphlet mailing group, and 10 percent for the visit group. One might conclude that the pamphlet failed to increase response to information that was spread through less direct (posters, for example) media. This seems analogous to the Bogota experiment in that PROFAMILIA had begun a radio campaign promoting the Centro Piloto clinic in February 1969, six months prior to the experiment. Neither the delivery of printed materials nor the visits of the family planning workers added to the stimulation already generated by the radio campaign and other informal sources of information.

A second study relevant to this topic is the early experiment by Reuben Hill, J. Mayone Stycos, and K. Back in Puerto Rico.[15] Similar to the Colombian study, the information campaign was conducted in a Latin American setting and was small-scale and of relatively short duration. Two methods of communication were employed—neighborhood group meetings and home delivery of pamphlets. Also similar to the Colombian experiment was the response in both communication methods. In contrast to the Bogota findings, however, the Puerto Rican study revealed significant (although not large) differences between approaches, with the group meeting being superior to home delivery of pamphlets. One possible interpretation of this is that personal influence and group pressure generated in discussions with groups of neighbors are more effective than impersonal influence of simple information transfer through the home delivery of the pamphlet materials.

In Bogota only impersonal methods of communication were used—a pamphlet is clearly impersonal, and a short visit by a previously unknown family planning worker is likely nearly as impersonal. The lack of significant differences between the pamphlet, home visit, and control groups in Bogota suggests that the PROFAMILIA radio campaign had created a knowledge-saturated population in that city prior to the experiment. Thus, most women in Bogota may have had some information about new clinic facilities prior to the experiment, and as a result neither the pamphlet nor the home visit added appreciably to the knowledge of the women contacted. From this point of view, adding a pamphlet or a home visit may have operated like another radio broadcast and would have been of limited motivational value.

The findings of all three studies support the view that adoption of new practices follows a sequence from awareness, information, and evaluation to trial and acceptance.[16] While mass media campaigns seem effective in taking people through awareness and information stages, several studies have shown that *personal* contact, in other words, influence from friends or relatives, becomes important at the evaluation and trial stages.[17] PROFAMILIA records for the period of the Bogota experiment show that roughly two-thirds of new patients cite friends, neighbors, and relatives as their source of information about the clinic. Moreover, it can be assumed that no matter how well they carried out their task, the family planning visitors were unable to establish the kind of personal contact one gets through friends or relatives.

The conclusion may be made that impersonal methods of communication tend to be similar to one another in their impact on the adoption of family planning because they are equally effective in creating awareness and relating minimal information about clinic services. In addition, an intensive widespread campaign involving various media, such as in Taiwan may increase community awareness and lower collective ignorance of family planning. In this way communication on family planning may increase among women and contribute to higher levels of response and clinic attendance than could be achieved with such directed media as pamphlets and home visits alone. At least for creating awareness, providing basic information, and arousing initial interest, mass media approaches such as radio campaigns that provide information to the community as a whole may be especially advantageous. This possibility will be further explained in the remainder of this chapter.

The Radio Campaign in Colombia

Prior to 1969 no large scale family planning information campaigns existed in Colombia. Groups and institutions interested in promoting family planning had arranged round-table discussions and other programs for radio designed to create a general awareness of population problems and to inform the well-educated minority about policy issues related to these problems. Opponents of family planning also expressed their views, and newspapers and other news media carried reports of the emerging debate.[18]

All of this certainly had some influence on the Colombian people's awareness of the population and birth control controversy, but its direct effect on their knowledge of clinic facilities and the details of contraceptive practice was certainly minimal. Communication efforts on these latter topics were restricted almost entirely to the PROFAMILIA speakers program where medical doctors associated with this organization addressed groups of union members or employees. Although several thousand people were contacted in this way prior to 1969, the campaign reached only a small proportion of the population.

The first mass campaign to bring new patients into the PROFAMILIA clinics began in mid-February 1969, and lasted until the end of November (or for a few radio stations, until mid-December) of the same year. At first there were nine radio stations broadcasting announcements in five different cities. Four of these stations were in Bogota, two in Barranquilla, and one each in Bucaramanga, Ibague, and Medellin. Each radio station broadcast twenty thirty-second announcements daily, telling women that family planning had many advantages and that information and assistance could be obtained in the local PROFAMILIA clinic. Later, in April, the number of stations was doubled as an additional radio station was added in Bogota, Barranquilla, Bucaramanga, and Ibague; two stations were added in Medellin; and one-station campaigns were inaugurated in Pereira, Manizales, and Armenia. Finally, in mid-June fifteen stations were introduced in new cities, bringing the total to thirty-three. The campaign ended when financial considerations forced PROFAMILIA to cut some of the stations and to reduce the number of announcements per day by one-half on the remaining stations. All announcements ended by December 15, 1969. The total cost of the campaign was estimated at $100,000, or about $10,000 for each month of operation.

A typical spot announcement went as follows:[19]

MAN: What will we do this year? John and Peter must continue in school. . . .

WOMAN: . . .And what about Beatrice, Lolita, and Manuel . . . it's years since they should have started (school) . . . Each year that goes by puts them further behind in their studies.

(Short stanza of music.)

ANNOUNCER 1: Avoid distress! Raise your children with foresight, love, and good judgment!

ANNOUNCER 2: Remember that parents should procreate with responsibility and not just reproduce!

ANNOUNCER 1: Children are the greatest treasure in a family. Each one deserves to be someone in life!

ANNOUNCER 2: Visit the family planning center at the PROFAMILIA clinic, in . . .(name of city) (address) . . . Service every day from . . . to . . .

Other announcements were similar, but the theme was always varied somewhat. Basically, women were advised to think carefully, to know how many children they could care for, to plan their family responsibly, to space their children scientifically, etc.; they were assured that PROFAMILIA could help them achieve the number of children they desired. The announcement always ended by advising the women to visit the local family planning center, at a given address, during specified hours. Only one clinic in each city was chosen for identification on the announcements, but only Bogota and Barranquilla have more than one clinic.

The overall influence of the radio campaign cannot be evaluated exclusively in terms of new patients entering the clinic, since some of the campaign's effects may have been equally important but less obvious. For example, a radio campaign may increase interest, discussion, and other forms of communication that may *eventually* lead to increased contraceptive practice. Simply knowing that a clinic exists may be an important step in the diffusion of family planning practice. Two surveys from Cali are relevant to these considerations, the first conducted two weeks prior to the Cali radio campaign, the other taken some four months after this campaign had started. The first survey will be referred to as the June (1969) study, the second as the September study. These surveys were taken for somewhat different purposes. The June survey was part of ASCOFAME's national fertility study.[20] It contains social background factors, a full contraceptive knowledge inventory, a fertility history,

Table V-6.   Selected Characteristics of Cali Women, by Education

	June Survey			September Survey		
	0-4 Years of School	5+ Years of School	All Women	0-4 Years of School	5+ Years of School	All Women[a]
Mean age of women	31.6	30.7	31.3	34.2	33.9	34.0
Percent currently mated	79	80	80	83	86	84
Mean number of living children	3.9	3.4	3.6	4.1	3.5	3.8
Percent Roman Catholic	93	96	94	96	96	96
Percent of women working	25	25	25	19	29	22
Percent who listen to radio announcements occasionally or "daily"	83	87	85	83	87	85
Number of cases	(121)	(81)	(201)	(151)	(252)	(403)

NOTE: Both groups contain only ever-mated fecund women aged 20-49.

[a] Weighted by age-education distribution of the June 1969 representative sample.

and a few questions on exposure to and knowledge from mass media. The September survey was carried out jointly by the Division of Socio-Demographic Studies at ASCOFAME and the Cornell University International Population Program.[21] It covered family planning communication, mass media, religion, and family structure. Some questions concerning family planning communication from the first survey were included in the second to facilitate comparisons.

The June data will first be analyzed to assess the influence of mass media on family planning knowledge and practice before the radio campaign; and the responses from the two surveys will be compared to assess changes in knowledge, attitudes, and practice that took place over the first four months of the campaign.

Because of certain differences between the two samples,[22] The analysis is focused on ever-mated women 20—49 years of age with at least one child, that is, on women who could most profitably use contraceptive information were it made available to them. In all comparisons education is controlled by showing characteristics of "high" and "low" education groups separately or by standardizing the September sample on the age-education distribution of the representative June sample.

Table V-6 shows the characteristics of the June and September samples for ever-mated women 20—49 years of age who have had at least one living child. While the September sample is slightly older (34.0 versus 31.3 years), on such characteristics as number of living children, religion, employment, marital status, and radio listening, the samples are quite similar.

Knowledge, Attitudes, and Practice
before the Radio Campaign

Regarding contraceptive knowledge, Table V-7 shows that slightly more than one-third of women in Cali prior to the radio campaign did not know that they could limit their fertility, and, when they were provided with the names of eleven common birth control methods, they were unable to recognize any method of birth control. An additional 1 percent knew that couples could limit fertility but were unable to name a method of birth control. While a majority knew some method of birth control, their range of knowledge was typically very limited—most could not name more than one or two methods. Of the total sample, only 14 percent were able to name three or more methods. The methods best known were the most modern ones, the contraceptive pill (74 percent) and the IUD (46 percent). Among more traditional methods the condom was best known (48 percent) while the douche was less well known (43 percent). Thirty-six percent had heard of rhythm, the only method approved by the Roman Catholic Church. All other methods were known by less than one-third of the women.

Regarding attitudes, Table V-7 indicates that in June, almost one-third of the Cali women sampled were negative or uncertain about birth control. Unfavorable women generally had less knowledge about birth control, hence in part their attitude may be taken as a reflection of their ignorance. · When asked why they were against birth control, a majority gave health reasons, although more than one-third gave religious or moral reasons. The precise nature of the health concern was not probed, but it seems likely that such probing would have revealed many erroneous assumptions.

Contraceptive practice among the sampled Cali women was determined from a series of questions regarding use of eleven common birth control methods (Table V-7). For each method the respondent was asked if she had ever heard of it, if she had ever used it, and if

Table V-7.   Responses to Family Planning Questions before Radio Campaign, All Cali Women Aged 15-49

Question	Answers	Percent Response
Do you know if there are things a man and his wife can do in order not to have children?	Yes	65
What things do you know that a man and his wife could do in order not to have children? (number of methods known)	None	35
	One	31
	Two	20
	More than three	14
Which of the following contraceptive methods do you know about?	Douche	43
	Withdrawal	28
	Rhythm	36
	Vaginal suppository	31
	Spermicidal cream or jelly	8
	Diaphragm	11
	Condom	48
	Intrauterine device (IUD)	46
	Anovulary pill	74
	Male sterilization	15
	Female sterilization	24
	Other method	6
Does use of such methods to avoid having children seem all right or not right to you?	Yes	70

she was using it at the time of the interview. For women who claimed they had or were using a method, distinction cannot be made between a single trial of a contraceptive and consistent practice over an extended period of time. However, because knowledge and use of each method was probed individually, and because women probably included single trials in their definition of prior use, the total who reported contraceptive practice is rather high. Fifty-five percent of ever-mated women in Cali claimed to have tried at least one method at some time.

To determine the possible impact of mass media on the awareness and knowledge of family planning, women were asked whether they had ever read anything about it in a newspaper, maga-

Why aren't you in agreement with the use of these methods? (for those against use of birth control)	Health	55
	Religious or moral	37
	Other	8
Have you or your spouse ever used a contraceptive method? (for ever-mated women with at least one child)	Yes	55
Have you ever heard a program over the radio discussing ways of avoiding unwanted pregnancies?	Yes	14
Do you know any written materials concerning how to avoid having unwanted children?	Yes	18
What is the principal written work you know? (to those who know some written materials)	Book	35
	Pamphlet or handout	15
	Magazine article	38
	Newspaper article	12
Did you read any part of this? How much did you read? (to those who know some written material)	None or leafed through	8
	One-half or less	27
	All	65
Number of cases		(383)

zine, or book. Only 14 percent of the women reported having heard a radio program on family planning, and only 18 percent having read something about it. (A majority of the readers had read the entire item, and the material was more likely to have appeared in some substantial publication, like a book or a magazine, than in a newspaper or pamphlet.) Only one in ten women reported ever having been to a meeting where methods of family planning were discussed.

Given the recency of the PROFAMILIA program, it is not surprising that only 27 percent knew a place where they might obtain family planning assistance. Of those who did know a place, however, the great majority knew the address also, although very few had

Table V-8. Birth Control Attitudes, Knowledge, and Practice before Radio Campaign, by Marital Status, Age, and Education

	Never-mated	Ever-mated			
		20-29	30-39	40-49	All Ages Ever-Mated
Percent who say the use of methods to avoid having children seems all right					
0-4 years of school	51	65	76	65	66
More than 4 years of school	77	90	92	88	90
All women	67	77	82	72	75
Percent who know at least one method of birth control					
0-4 years of school	48	73	94	84	83
More than 4 years of school	77	95	97	83	94
All women	66	85	95	84	89
Mean number of methods known (for those who know at least one method of birth control)					
0-4 years of school	1.9	3.6	4.3	4.2	4.3
More than 4 years of school	3.4	6.4	5.6	5.1	5.4
All women	3.0	4.9	4.7	4.5	4.8
Percent who have used a birth control method					
0-4 years of school		36	50	52	45
More than 4 years of school		76	73	58	76
All women		54	62	54	57
Percent who know a place where they teach women how to avoid having unwanted children					
0-4 years of school	3	16	38	27	27
More than 4 years of school	2	28	31	18	28
All women	3	22	35	24	27
Number of cases					
0-4 years of school	(29)	(48)	(48)	(25)	(121)
More than 4 years of school	(48)	(41)	(29)	(12)	(82)
All women	(77)	(89)	(77)	(37)	(203)

SOURCE: Representative sample of 383 women aged 15-49 years, Cali, June 1969.

ever been there. Thus, the conclusion may be made that for the period immediately prior to the radio campaign in Cali, neither clinic facilities nor mass media were critical factors in the diffusion of family planning.

Controlling for education, age, and marital experience in the pre-campaign Cali sample, the better educated women and women with some fertility experience were found to be more positive to family planning, more knowledgeable about contraceptive methods, and better informed on the location of family planning services (Table V-8). Young unmarried women in particular had low levels of knowledge about methods and services, as one might expect given the low saliency of these issues for them. Among the ever-mated women with children, the influence of age is uncertain since there is considerable variation in age patterns from one variable to another and from one educational group to another. Nevertheless, young, better educated women were clearly most favorable to family planning and most knowledgeable about contraceptive methods, while less educated women age 30 — 39 years were best informed on available clinic services. This latter finding seems congruent with the economic and fertility status of less educated women, 30 — 39 years of age. These women were relatively ignorant of and unfamiliar with contraceptive methods; they had relatively limited access to private medical services; and they may have had several children already, yet they faced the prospects of more children in their remaining fertile years. It could be argued that they were relatively well informed because they were the women who had the greatest need for public family planning clinic facilities. Yet even in this relatively well-informed and apparently interested class of women, only a minority (38 percent) were aware of the location of any clinic facilities prior to the campaign.

Before turning to an analysis of the influence of the radio campaign on the distribution of information about family planning and clinic facilities, brief note should be made of the extent to which radio had penetrated into the daily lives of Colombian women. Table V-9 shows that prior to the campaign almost all women in the Cali sample listened to the radio occasionally, and a majority listened daily. While the proportion who never read newspapers (13 percent) is similar to the proportion who never listened to radio (14 percent), only about one-third read newspapers daily. Table V-10 indicates that schooling is closely related to newspaper reading but not related to radio listening. Indeed, radio listening and newspaper reading are largely independent activities. Unlike newspaper read-

Table V-9.   Exposure to Radio Announcements,
Newspapers, and Magazines before
Radio Campaign (in percent)

	Never	Occasionally	Daily	Total
Listen to radio anouncements	14	20	66	100
Read newspapers	13	50	37	100
Read magazines	27	47	26	100

SOURCE: Representative sample of 383 women aged 15-49 years, Cali, June 1969.

ing, radio is likely to reach women of all ages and levels of education. Since the better educated women were already better informed on contraceptive matters, a good way to reach the less educated women may be through radio.

Knowledge, Attitudes, and Practice in Cali after the Radio Information Campaign

The respondents in the pre-campaign Cali June survey were asked: "Have you ever heard a program over the radio discussing ways of avoiding unwanted pregnancies?" While there had been no advertisements explicitly encouraging people to go to family planning clinics prior to the campaign, it is apparent that the topic of family planning had occasionally been dealt with in various women's radio programs and round-table discussions of one kind and another, for 14 percent of all the women in the June survey claimed to have heard such a program (Table V-7). If only ever-mated women, age 20 - 49 years, with at least one child are considered, the proportion who had heard such a program prior to the campaign rises to 18 percent (Table V-11). Women with less schooling were more likely to have heard a radio program on family planning by June. Whether this is due to the type of program that less educated women listened to or to their sensitivity to the issue is not clear.

The respondents in the second Cali survey (September), taken roughly four months after the campaign started, were asked: "Have you ever heard a (radio) announcement concerning family planning services?" A rough estimate can be made of the proportion who heard an announcement over the first four months of the campaign by comparing the percent who admitted hearing an announcement in September with the percent who had heard one in June. In mak-

Table V-10.   Knowledge and Use of Contraception
before Radio Campaign, by Exposure
to Mass Media Materials on Family Planning

	Has Heard a Radio Program on Family Planning		Knows Written Materials on Family Planning	
	Yes	No	Yes	No
Percent who know a place where they teach women to avoid unwanted children				
0-4 years of school	26	25	44	23
More than 4 years of school	40	22	39	21
All women	32	24	40	22
Mean number of contraceptive methods known				
0-4 years of school	3.6	3.3	4.8	3.2
More than 4 years of school	6.1	5.7	7.7	5.1
All women	4.6	4.2	5.1	3.8
Percent who have used birth control at least once				
0-4 years of school	43	45	44	45
More than 4 years of school	73	74	87	69
All women	54	57	74	53

NOTE: Sample includes ever-mated fecund women aged 20-49 years, Cali, June 1969.

ing this comparison one should note that the June question is less specific than the September one, which asks about having heard programs on *family planning* services. While this difference is slight, it may underestimate somewhat the proportion who had heard a radio announcement during the period of the campaign. It should also be noted that in both surveys the concept "family planning" was not defined prior to asking this question, thus increasing comparability between the surveys.

From one survey to another, the proportion of fertile women who had heard something about family planning on the radio increases dramatically from 18 to 71 percent (Table V-11). The greatest increase occurred among young women with higher education, both because few of these women had heard anything prior to the campaign, and because during the campaign they were by far the most exposed to the announcement. Perhaps most important, however, is the fact that the proportion who heard the announcement is high (between 60 and 80 percent) for both young and old, better and less educated. Thus, radio appears to democratize exposure to information. There is only a slight tendency for the younger, better educated (who initially had more family planning information) to be more exposed to the announcement.

While those who heard something do not differ from those who did not with regard to schooling, labor force status, family size, and age, they differ in their radio listening habits. In both surveys, the women who heard an advertisement or program were more likely to be daily radio listeners and to have a radio in their homes (Table V-12). Those who heard the announcement after the campaign were not only more likely to listen to the radio, but because of this they were also more likely to have heard announcements for other pro-

Table V-11.   Percent Who Said They Had Heard an Announcement or Program on Family Planning over the Radio, June and September 1969, by Age and Education

| | Schooling Completed | | |
	0-4 years	5+ years	All Women
Before campaign (June 1969)			
Women aged 20-29	23	6	18
Women aged 30-39	23	9	20
Women aged 40-49	18	—[a]	18
All women aged 20-49	22	6	18
After campaign (September 1969)			
Women aged 20-29	60	81	72
Women aged 30-39	71	70	70
Women aged 40-49	71	69	70
All women aged 20-49	66	74	71
Percent change between June and September			
Women aged 20-29	37	75	54
Women aged 30-39	48	61	50
Women aged 40-49	53	—[a]	53
All women aged 20-49	44	68	53

NOTE: Sample includes ever-mated fecund women aged 20-49 years.
[a] Less than ten cases.

ducts or services. Thus, as indicated in Table V-12, women who claimed to have heard a radio announcement on family planning services were also more likely to have heard announcements for other commonly advertised products, such as Elephant Soap, Red Skin cigarettes, and public vaccination. These findings do not appear to be the result of a tendency for some respondents to falsely claim to have heard all announcements about which they were questioned; for the proportion who claimed to have heard radio announcements for certain non-existent products (such as Zipa Soap, Tequendama Oil, and Green River cigarettes—names that were fabricated to test for response bias) was no higher among those who

Table V-12.   Selected Characteristics, by Exposure to Radio Announcements on Family Planning, June and September 1969

	June Survey			September Survey[a]		
	Heard Message	Did Not Hear	Total	Heard Message	Did Not Hear	Total
Mean number of years of schooling	4.2	4.2	4.2	5.8	5.6	5.7
Percent now working	24	28	27	26	29	28
Mean number of living children	3.4	3.5	3.5	3.8	3.8	3.8
Mean age	32.2	32.2	32.2	—	—	—
Percent who listen to announcements over the radio daily	74	52	55	68	44	62
Percent who have radios	—	—	—	97	85	94
Percent heard announcement (possible) on:						
Elephant Soap	—	—	—	79	52	68
Public Vaccination	—	—	—	69	44	62
Red Skin Cigarettes	—	—	—	90	59	82
Percent heard announcement (impossible) on:						
Zipa Soap	—	—	—	14	8	13
Tequendama Oil	—	—	—	16	12	15
Green River Cigarettes	—	—	—	12	6	5
Number of cases	(50)	(321)	(371)	(311)	(113)	(424)

NOTE: Sample includes ever-mated fecund women aged 20-49 years.
[a]   September figures weighted by age-education distribution of representative June survey.

claimed to have heard the family planning announcement than among those who claimed not to have heard it.[23]

Learning the Meaning of Family Planning

What did the Cali women who heard the radio announcements on family planning learn? The term family planning is a common euphemism for birth control, which is prone to misinterpretation even in nations where its use is long established. In many parts of Latin America the term is more recent, and it is sometimes used to include activities that promote the education, health, and well-being of one's children. For many people, the radio announcements may have provided a first exposure to the central meaning of the term "planificación familiar," since they specifically referred to it in the context of "not having more children than one can support and educate well."

In the September survey the open-ended question was asked: "What do you think family planning is?" The responses were put into three categories: "Do not know"; "To do with the health and education of one's children"; and "Concerning family size, spacing, or contraceptive practice." Then the women were asked two more specific questions: "Does family planning have more to do with the necessities of one's home or with the size of one's family?" and "Does family planning have more to do with the health of one's children or with the number of children that one has?"

Seventy-eight percent of ever-mated women with at least one living child knew the correct answer to the initial open-ended question (Table V-13). While 90 percent of those with five or more years of schooling were able to answer the question correctly, only 61 percent of those with less schooling were able to do so. Younger women also more frequently had correct answers. Most important for an hypothesis, however, is the finding that having heard the radio announcement is predictive of knowledge—84 percent of those women who heard the announcement (but only one-half the women who had not) gave a correct definition.

The direction of causation in the association between hearing and understanding the message is somewhat problematic. While women who heard the announcement may have learned about family planning, women who knew the definition may have been more likely to understand the announcement and remember that they had heard it. Of these two possibilities, the data lend more support to the first. Among the better educated, 91 percent of those who had heard the announcement gave a correct answer, as compared with 73 percent among those who had not. Among the less educated women the difference was much more marked: 82 percent gave a correct answer among those who had heard, 34 percent among those who had not. Thus, the better educated women knew what family planning is whether or not they had heard the announcement, while the less educated, being initially unfamiliar with the concept, learned most from the announcement.

Table V-14 shows that correct answers to the more specific questions on family planning were also more prevalent among those who heard the announcement. These questions reveal some confusion with the term family planning. When asked whether family planning has more to do with the necessities of one's home or with the number of children one has, 27 percent answered "both are equally correct," while 34 percent said "necessities of home" was most correct. Twelve percent could not answer at all. Only one-quarter of the women felt that family planning was principally concerned with family size. While the great majority of women who heard the announcement understood what family planning was and what the intent of the message was, they may not have picked up

Table V-13. Percent Who Know What Family Planning Is after the Campaign, by Age, Education, and Exposure to Radio Announcements on Family Planning

	Age			All Women
Heard announcement	20-29	30-39	40-49	Aged 20-49
0-4 years of school	80	67	68	82
More than 4 years of school	94	92	78	91
All women	90	84	76	84
Did not hear announcement				
0-4 years of school	35	35	22	34
More than 4 years of school	76	80	62	73
All women	53	61	44	54
All Women				
0-4 years of school	67	57	57	61
More than 4 years of school	93	91	79	90
All women	83	80	75	78

NOTE: Sample includes ever-mated fecund women aged 20-49 years, September 1969.

Table V-14.   Percent Who Knew, after Radio Campaign, That Family Planning Concerned Size of Family, by Exposure to Radio Announcement

Family planning has more to do with necessities of home or size of family?	Did Not Hear Announcement	Heard Announcement	All Women
Could not answer	5	32	12
Necessities of home	36	28	34
Size of family	29	20	27
Both equally	30	20	27
Total	100	100	100
Number of cases	(329)	(108)	(437)
Family planning has more to do with health of children or size of family?			
Could not answer	43	59	48
Health	8	6	6
Size of family	36	18	32
Both equally	14	17	14
Total	100	100	100
Number of cases	(329)	(108)	(437)

NOTE: Sample includes ever-mated fecund women aged 20-49 years, September 1969.

the directive concerning precisely where to go for services. Accordingly, women who heard the announcement were asked: "Where did (it) . . . tell you to go? To a health clinic or to a drug store?" Close to three-quarters of the women with at least one living child could not remember, and virtually all the others said "health center." This would suggest that women did not remember the announcement in any detail, though such details may be less important than the general information they gained.

Learning about Clinic Facilities
Questions concerning the existence and address of clinic facilities were asked in both the June and September surveys. In the June survey respondents were asked, "Do you know any place where they teach women how to avoid (unwanted) pregnancies?" and in Sep-

tember, "Have you heard about a health center, or medical office in this city called PROFAMILIA?" In both surveys those who knew of a clinic were asked if they knew the address. Results of the September survey are shown in Table V-15 (See Table V-8 for June survey.)

The questions on clinic facilities in the two surveys are not directly comparable, for the question in the June survey refers to *any place* where family planning services may be sought, while the September survey refers specifically to PROFAMILIA. Knowledge of PROFAMILIA in the second survey may understate the overall level of knowledge since some women may have known about government clinics, but not specifically PROFAMILIA clinics, where family planning clinic services are offered. Despite this bias, however, knowledge of PROFAMILIA clinics was much greater in September 1969 (44 percent) than knowledge of *all* places where family planning services could be sought in June (only 27 percent). Similarly, while only 27 percent of women aged 20—49 years with at least one child knew the address of *any* clinic in June (Table V-8), 33 percent knew the address of PROFAMILIA's clinic in September. Increases in knowledge are much greater among the younger women and, to a lesser extent, among those with higher education.

Contraceptive Practice

If awareness of clinic facilities increased, was it followed by action? Between June and September 1969, 150 to 250 new patients went to the Cali PROFAMILIA clinic each month. In a city with roughly 120,000 mated women of child-bearing age, this number of new patients does not suggest a significant impact on clinical services. Certainly some of the women would go to the clinic even in the absence of a radio campaign; hence the influence of the radio campaign would appear to have been very small.

It is possible, of course, that the campaign affected the use of birth control more generally, that is, outside of clinic methods. Unfortunately, differences in question wording in the two samples prevent determination of the increase in contraceptive practice from June to September.[24] However, since the September survey asked women who had ever used contraceptives when they began to do so, it is possible to estimate the percent of ever-users who began to practice birth control in the previous six months, the period corresponding roughly to the expansion and promotion of the PROFAMILIA clinic. As may be seen in Table V-16, the proportion of women who began in the six months prior to September is rather

Table V-15. Percent Who Knew of Existence and Address of Family Planning Clinic Facilities, by Age and Education

| | Schooling Completed | | |
	0-4 years	5+ years	All Women
Knew of the PROFAMILIA clinic, September 1969[a]			
Women aged 20-29	52	59	56
Women aged 30-39	35	47	43
Women aged 40-49	33	28	30
All women aged 20-49	40	46	44
Change in percent between June and September 1969 of those who knew of a clinic[b]			
Women aged 20-29	+36	+31	+34
Women aged 30-39	-3	+16	+8
Women aged 40-49	+ 6	+10	+6
All women aged 20-49	+13	+18	+17
Knew address of PROFAMILIA clinic, September 1969[a]			
Women aged 20-29	35	44	41
Women aged 30-39	35	36	32
Women aged 40-49	25	20	22
All women aged 20-49	29	35	33
Change in percent between June and September 1969 of those who knew address of a clinic[b]			
Women aged 20-29	+19	+16	+19
Women aged 30-39	-3	+5	-3
Women aged 40-49	-2	+2	-2
All women aged 20-49	+2	+7	+6

NOTE: Sample includes ever-mated fecund women aged 20-49 years.

[a]   Samples for the September 1969 survey are weighted by the age-education distribution of women in the representative June 1969 survey to allow direct comparisons between the two samples.

[b]   Difference between percent who knew of (or knew the address of) any clinic where people are taught to avoid pregnancies in June 1969 (see Table V-8) and the percent who knew of (or the address of) PROFAMILIA in September 1969 (this table).

Table V-16. Birth Control Use, by Age and Education

	Age			
	20-29	30-39	40-49	All Women Aged 20-49[a]
Percent who have ever used birth control				
0-4 years of school	31	16	18	62
More than 4 years of school	66	70	27	22
All women	48	37	21	39
Percent of ever-users who began use in six months prior to survey, September 1969				
0-4 years of school	27	15	12	15
More than 4 years of school	13	13	6	15
All women	23	8	10	15

NOTE: Sample includes ever-mated fecund women aged 20-49 years.

[a] Total weighted by age-education distribution of the representative June 1969 survey.

high, especially among less educated women aged 20—29 years—27 percent of those who admitted ever using family planning began use in this period. Thus, relatively low levels of current use among the less educated young women contrasts with the high proportion of these users who began contraceptive practice very recently. Among the better educated young women, whose use was higher to begin with, most women began use prior to the campaign and the opening of clinic services. It would appear that many young, less educated women have recently been influenced to begin family planning. The major part of this increase can be attributed directly to the PROFAMILIA or other clinics, since 55 percent of women who began practice in the prior six months did so after attending a clinic. However, since 45 percent of the recent adopters had never attended a clinic, some of the influence of the campaign may have been indirect, operating through increased private awareness about family planning.

Other Sources of Information: Written Material and Word of Mouth

One indicator of changing awareness and concern might be an increase in the proportion of women who have read something on birth control. The June survey asked: "Do you know any written materials concerning the way to avoid having (too many) children?" The September survey asked: "Have you read anything concerning family planning or how not to have too many children?" The proportion who had read something almost doubled from 17 percent in June to 31 percent in September (Table V-17). The increase was greatest among better educated women despite the fact that they were no more knowledgeable of written materials to begin with. Over one-half of the women 20 —29 years of age with five years or more schooling had read something by the time of the September survey, while only one-third had done so in June. Either there have been recent substantial increases in the production of printed materials on family planning in Cali, or, as seems more likely, the radio campaign heightened interest in existing materials.

Word-of-mouth communication may also play an important role in the diffusion of contraceptive knowledge and birth planning. Three questions asked in September are pertinent: "Have you ever talked to anyone about family planning?" "Who was the last person

Table V-17. Percent Who Had Read Something on Family Planning, by Age and Education, June and September 1969

	Age 20-29	30-39	40-49	All Women Aged 20-49[a]
Before the campaign, June 1969				
0-4 years of school	7	7	14	8
More than 4 years of school	33	28	18	29
All women	19	15	15	17
After the campaign, September 1969				
0-4 years of school	19	21	16	19
More than 4 years of school	53	49	31	49
All women	35	32	21	31
Increase, June to September				
0-4 years of school	12	14	2	11
More than 4 years of school	20	21	13	20
All women	16	17	6	14

NOTE: Sample includes ever-mated fecund women aged 20-49 years.
[a] Totals for September 1969 weighted by age-education distribution of the representative June 1969 survey.

you talked with?" "How frequently do you discuss family size problems with your husband?" One-half of the fertile women aged 20—49 years claimed to have talked to someone, and almost three-fourths of the younger, better educated had done so. When asked who they had last spoken with, just over one-half said "friends" or "relatives," 20 percent said "spouse" and 23 percent said "medical doctors." One-fifth had never discussed family planning with their husbands while one-third had discussed it "frequently." To what extent this reasonably high incidence of discussion is due to the radio campaign is not known, but it is clear that the last two months of the campaign operated in the context of very high general awareness. If not at the beginning of the campaign, then certainly toward the end, the Cali women of the sample were talking and reading about family planning to a considerable extent. It is most likely that new information about the existence of the PRO-FAMILIA clinic, which was spread widely by radio, also became part of discussions between women, their friends, relatives, and husbands.

Community Difference in Response to the Radio Campaign: Cali, Armero, and Cucuta

In describing the pattern of family planning communication in Cali, it must be remembered that this large city may not be typical. Since more of PROFAMILIA's efforts are currently directed at smaller cities, an examination was made of the results of the September survey in Cucuta (1964 population 137,000) and Armero (1964 population 17,500). The same sampling procedure utilized in the September Cali survey was also followed in these smaller communities, hence the overall results of these studies may be directly compared.

In each of the communities a PROFAMILIA clinic had opened somewhat prior to the radio campaign. Radio announcements began on June 1, 1969, and ended in early December of the same year. The number of radio stations contracted for the campaign varied roughly with the size of the community—Cali had four stations, Cucuta three, and Armero one. As Table V-18 indicates, radio listening characteristics in each community are directly related to the size of the community. As community size increases, a higher proportion of women had radios, a higher proportion of women listened to their radios daily, and a higher proportion had heard commonly advertised products (for example, Elephant Soap). The percent who claimed to have heard an advertisement on a fictitious product (for example, Zipa Soap) varies in no clear way with community size.

Differences in the percent who heard the announcements on family planning are also not directly related to community size, for the proportion is lowest in Cucuta, where women are also *least* likely to know what family planning means, least likely to have read something on family planning, and least likely to have spoken to their husbands about this topic. For example, only 17 percent of the women in Cucuta had spoken to their husbands about family planning, while roughly twice this proportion had done so in Cali and Armero. These results suggest that there may be some dimensions of traditionalism in these communities that are independent of community size.

Whereas Cali is considered to be a progressive city, Cucuta is a traditional city close to the Venezuelan border, isolated from the principal cultural centers of Colombia. The area around Cucuta continues to be dominated by coffee agriculture, and the people are said to reflect this in traditional values and practices. Armero, while small, is at the northern edge of Tolima, within the web of

Table V-18. Selected Aspects of Family Planning Communication and Traditionalism in Cali, Cucuta, and Armero (in percent)

	Cali	Cucuta	Armero
Have a radio	93	92	89
Listen to radio announcements daily	61	56	50
Heard advertisement on Elephant Soap (possible)	24	19	14
Heard advertisement on Zipa Soap (impossible)	13	16	20
Heard announcement on family planning	70	43	63
Could correctly define family planning	63	43	50
Have read something on family planning	36	21	32
Talk to husband frequently about family planning	33	17	34
Go to communion weekly	8	15	11
Do not approve of any changes in the Roman Catholic Church	30	57	54
Believe one should have all children that God sends	10	26	19
Number of cases	(445)	(355)	(178)

NOTE: Based on all ever-mated women sampled in these communities, September 1969.

influence of both Ibague and Bogota. Contact with these large cities is substantial and may influence the attitudes of the people who live there. Thus, of the three communities, Cucuta may be the most traditional. Table V-18 shows that a higher percent of women in Cucuta go to communion weekly, do not approve of changes in the Roman Catholic Church, and believe that one should have all the children God sends. In general, women in Cali are most liberal about these issues, and women in Armero fall between.

It would appear that the general ambience concerning family planning may be closely related to wider patterns of traditionalism in a community and is only partially related to the structure of mass media like radio. The percent of women sampled in the three cities who claim to have heard the PROFAMILIA announcement on family planning over radio or to have read something on family planning seems to reflect the traditionalism in the three communities. While radio announcements may serve to break down these traditional barriers, the barriers may nevertheless prevent the announcements or other forms of propaganda from having any major impact on family planning practices for some time to come. This hypothesis may be tested in part by analyzing the pattern of response to radio campaigns in communities of various size and traditionalism.

The Influence of the Radio Campaign on Clinic Attendance

In Cali, as previously pointed out, overall levels of clinic attendance over the period of the radio campaign did increase substantially at least for young, less educated women. Moreover, general levels of awareness and discussion of family planning issues appear to have increased substantially over the period of the campaign. These findings suggest that many of the new patients went to the Cali clinic over this period because of the radio announcements, but how many would have gone to the clinic in the absence of the radio campaign cannot be determined. The Cali clinic was established just prior to the beginning of the campaign, hence no trend line had been established. To analyze the influence of the radio program on clinic attendance, longer established clinics, whose pattern of growth prior to the campaign can be determined, will be considered.

The Numerical Response

If the advertising program was truly effective, a rise in the number of new patients could be expected immediately after the beginning of the announcements and a leveling off, or perhaps a decline, in new patients sometime after they were discontinued. Figure V-1 showed that the number of new patients did rise sharply after the onset of the campaign and began declining soon after it ended. The possible influence of the radio, however, may be obscured by other factors. At least three alternative explanations must be eliminated before a causal link can be be posited between the campaign and the growth of the clinic population.

First, in several instances, clinics were opened either somewhat before or just after initiation of the radio campaign. Thus, the rapid increases and declines in new patients among such clinics may to some extent reflect only the natural pattern of growth, leveling off, and decline shown in Figure V-2 and Figure V-3.

Secondly, the rise and decline in numbers of patients may have been due to extraneous influences such as shifts in public opinion unrelated to the radio campaign.

Thirdly, variations in numbers of new patients may also be *seasonal*. Clinic personnel have noted high levels of new patient intake in January through October and much lower levels around December. Unfortunately the natural monthly trend of rise and decline corresponds closely to the onset and cessation of the campaign, hence increases in patients during the campaign could be partially due to seasonal fluctuations.

To control for these three alternative explanations, the following methodology was developed. First, a trend line representing clinic growth in the period prior to the campaign was calculated for each clinic. This trend line was calculated as the linear regression line ($y = ax + b$) for the six-month period from August 1968 to January 1969. This period spans the December slump in new patients and thereby avoids being seriously influenced by seasonal patterns. (While this six months reflects the trend just prior to the campaign, the choice of six months rather than a longer period turns out to be somewhat arbitrary. The principal cities to be considered have been established for some time, and their trend lines for the six-month period indicated are scarcely different from the trend lines for one year or more.) Second, the trend line for each clinic was projected into the future to yield an estimate of the number of new patients that would have been expected over the campaign period in the absence of radio announcements or other influences. By comparing the expected number with the actual, the effects of new sources of influence (such as the radio announcements) coming into operation during the campaign can be estimated. Third, to determine whether observed effects are actually due to the radio campaign and not to unknown influences operating in the same period, clinics that were announced in the campaign were compared with clinics in the same cities that were not announced. If the radio announcements were effective, increases in new patients could be expected above the trend line only in those clinics that were announced. The clinics that were not announced should have continued to follow the trend line.

Two of the largest and longest-established Bogota clinics, Centro Piloto and Hospital San José, reached their peaks several years ago and have had long histories of rather constant negative growth rates since then. Figure V-4 shows the projection of trends in new patients for these clinics into the period of the campaign. These trend lines indicate a decided downward trend for Centro Piloto and a slight downward trend for San José. Figure V-4 also shows the number of women who went to the two clinics during and slightly after the campaign. The contrast is striking between Centro Piloto, which was identified by the radio program, and San José, which was not. While San José continued to follow the trend line until December (when it dropped lower, perhaps following the seasonal pattern) Centro Piloto dramatically reversed its downward trend immediately after the campaign began so that the number of new patients rose markedly each month until October. At the peak period, the number of new patients in Centro Piloto was nearly four times what it would have been if the trend prior to the campaign had continued. In November and December the number of new patients declined somewhat from the October peak but still remained far above the level prior to the campaign.

The same statistical procedure was followed for two clinics in Barranquilla, one of which (Atlantico) was announced over the radio, while the other (Bautista) was not (Figure V-5). In contrast to the Bogota clinics, these clinics were experiencing pre-campaign growth: slow growth for Bautista, rapid for Atlantico. While the growth trend in the Barranquilla clinics contrasts with the decline trend in Bogota, the reaction to radio advertising appears to have been similar in both cities. The Bautista clinic's progressive inflow continued to parallel the trend line, reflecting the fact that it was not announced over the radio, and the Atlantico clinic, which was announced, experienced an inflow substantially beyond expectation. Thus, even during its natural period of rapid growth, a clinic's rate of expansion can be accelerated by radio announcements. After the campaign, the inflow to Atlantico dropped somewhat but it still remained above what could have been expected from the pre-campaign trend. As was seen with the Centro Piloto clinic, the influence of radio appears to continue for some time after the campaign.

Since no other cities had more than one PROFAMILIA clinic functioning during the radio campaign, no further comparisons between announced and unannounced clinics are possible. However, campaign impact on those clinics that had established discernible trends in growth or decline prior to the campaign can be examined. A

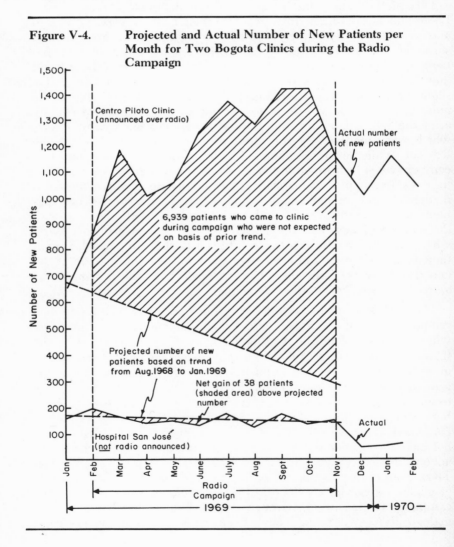

Figure V-4.   Projected and Actual Number of New Patients per Month for Two Bogota Clinics during the Radio Campaign

good example is provided by Medellin, which like the other larger, older clinics in Bogota, was experiencing a steady downward trend in new patients prior to the campaign (Figure V-2). As in Bogota and Barranquilla, the campaign in Medellin seems to have reversed this trend (Figure V-6). The reversal appears to have been temporary however, for following the campaign the number of new patients fell to the levels that had existed earlier.

Given that clinic growth fluctuates rapidly in the first year of operation, eighteen months seem generally necessary before a stable

Figure V-5.   **Projected and Actual Number of New Patients per Month for Two Barranquilla Clinics during the Radio Campaign**

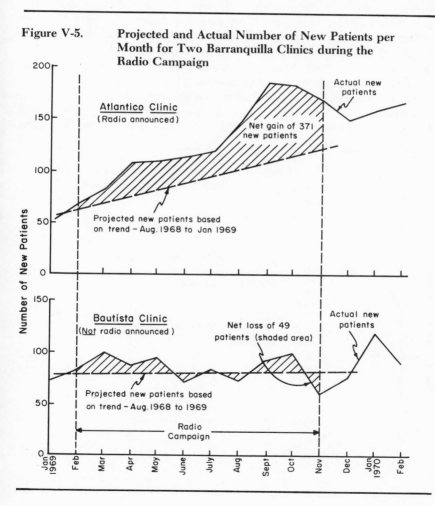

linear trend can be discerned. The only other clinics in operation long enough to permit a trend analysis, then, are in Pasto, Cucuta, Buenaventura, and Sogamoso, all cities with less than 250,000 inhabitants. According to the hypothesis that the number of new patients "naturally" begins to decline after some two years of clinic operation, all these clinics were facing imminent declines. While Figure V-7 shows that the pattern varies somewhat from city to city, none of these clinics seems to have responded to the radio campaign in the way that the larger, older clinics in the big cities did. Cucuta, Buenaventura, and Sogamoso followed the trend line until the termination of the campaign, then dropped below the line. Pasto is similar except that it dropped well below the trend line by the middle of the campaign. It would appear that the radio programs in the smaller cities may have, at best, served to postpone the transition from positive to negative rates of increase.

The information campaign in the smaller cities, if effective at all, was certainly less effective than in the larger cities. Table V-19 shows for each clinic the percent of new patients over the campaign

Figure V-6.   Projected and actual Number of New Patients per Month for the Medellin Clinic during the Radio Campaign

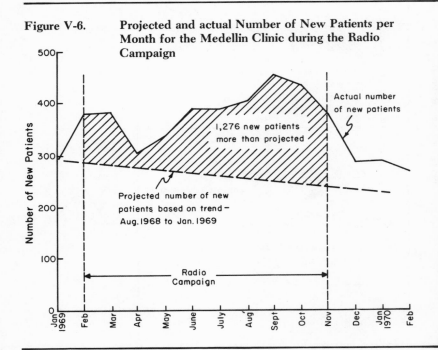

period who were unexpected on the basis of the trend prior to the campaign. The larger the city (and the larger the clinic), the greater the impact of the campaign. Not only did Centro Piloto accept the greatest absolute number of new patients, but this number was largest relative to its total intake, comprising a surprising 57 percent. The

Figure V-7.   Projected and Actual Number of New Patients per Month for Clinics in Pasto, Cucuta, Buenaventura, and Sogamoso during the Radio Campaign

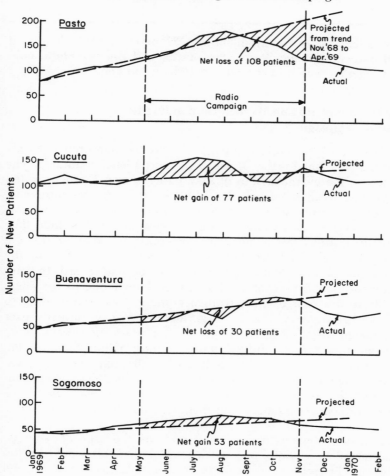

**Table V-19.   Unexpected New Patients at Selected Clinics over
Period of the 1969 Radio Campaign**

	Total New Patients	Number Unexpected	Percent Unexpected
Centro Piloto (Bogota)	12,044	6,939	57
Medellin	3,866	1,276	32
Atlantico (Barranquilla)	1,295	371	28
Cucuta, Pasto, Sogamoso, Buenaventura (combined)	765	0	0

corresponding figure for Medellin was 32 percent; for Atlantico it
was 28 percent. Cucuta, Pasto, Sogamoso, and Buenaventura, considered together, had no net gain above the trend line.

Characteristics of Bogota Women Responding to the Radio Campaign

The influence of the radio campaign should be measured not only
by the quantity but by the "quality" of the patients it attracts. The
influence on the characteristics of new patients may be investigated
through data available from the PROFAMILIA intake interview,
which gathers information on several socio-demographic characteristics and on how the woman came to know about the clinic. For
the month of July 1969 a question concerning whether or not the
new patient had heard the radio announcement was added to the
interview at Centro Piloto. While 54 percent had heard the announcement, only 5 percent attributed their knowledge of the clinic
primarily to this source; most women credited their information to
friends and relatives. Given the large increase in new patients after
the campaign began, it appears that the radio announcements were
at least an important secondary source of information. Some of the
radio's influence may have been mediated through personal communication among friends. Many women who had had vague no-
tions about the existence of clinic facilities from friends may have
learned more concrete facts about them through the radio announcements.

   If the announcements had any influence on the type of new patient attracted to a clinic, one would expect that this would be de-
tectable in differences between those who claimed they learned
about the clinic through the radio announcements and those who

Table V-20. Selected Characteristics of New Centro Piloto Clinic Patients in July 1969, by Exposure to Radio Announcement

	Heard Radio Announcement	Learned about Clinic through Announcement	All Women
Mean age	28.0	28.3	27.9
Percent with			
no schooling	6	8	5
1-3 years of school	33	40	35
4-6 years of school	35	26	33
more than 6 years of school	26	26	27
Percent with			
1-2 living children	30	18	30
3-4 living children	36	30	38
more than 4 living children	34	52	32
Percent who had practiced contraception previously	12	24	12
Percent who have radio in home	96	100	91
Number of cases	(422)	(39)	(789)

SOURCE: Intake interviews with new patients registering at the Centro Piloto clinic in July 1969.

claimed they learned about it through other sources. Table V-20 compares characteristics of women who had heard the radio announcements and women who attributed their knowledge of the clinic to the radio announcements with the characteristics of the clinic population as a whole for the month of July 1969. While women who learned about the clinic through the radio announcements are somewhat older than the clinic population as a whole, this difference is very small. Similarly, educational differences are slight, though there is some suggestion that those who learned about the clinic over the radio are somewhat less educated than the general clinic population. The differences are more pronounced for number of living children, previous contraceptive practice, and possession of a radio. Women who learned about the clinic through the radio announcements are twice as likely to have practiced contraception previously; and they are of relatively high parity, the majority having five or more children. One gets the impression that these women comprise a small, highly motivated minority, many of whom have had unsatisfactory experiences with contraception leading them to the clinic for assistance.

Relative Cost of Radio Campaigns

The cost of the Colombian radio campaign is best considered in relative terms—how much does it cost to attract a new patient through a radio campaign relative to the cost of attracting a new patient through other methods of communication? On the basis of the communication experiment, a cost estimate can be made for each new patient added through home visit or through delivery of pamphlet material. Very roughly (since the experiment was very short-term and did not present a precise picture of costs for a longer-term project), enumerating a population to determine "eligible" women would cost about thirty cents (five Colombian pesos) per eligible woman found. Delivery of pamphlet material would cost another fifteen cents per woman, while actually visiting the woman would cost at least sixty cents (ten pesos). Without a concurrent radio campaign, but with careful selection so that about 30 percent of those women actually enumerated would be approached, and with better motivation techniques, the difference in response between those who receive and those who do not receive the communications might under most optimistic conditions rise to a 6 percent response for pamphlets to a 10 percent response for home visits. Even under these optimal conditions, the total cost per new patient attracted in the pamphlet approach would be about $7.50 and for the home visit would be about $9.00. Conversely, if the return was closer to that actually found in Taiwan, the cost per new patient would be at least twice this. If the return was similar to that found in the Bogota study, the cost per patient would be at least four times higher—$30.00 per patient for pamphlet and $36.00 per patient for home visit. How do the costs of the radio campaign compare with these crude estimates for pamphlet and home visit?

The ten-month PROFAMILIA radio campaign of 1969 cost roughly $100,000, but this cost was not distributed equally between radio stations and was much less equally distributed between cities. Bogota not only had more stations broadcasting (five at the peak of the campaign), but the cost per announcement over these stations was higher than in other cities. For an extended campaign of twenty one-half-minute announcements over several months, cost per month in Bogota ranged from roughly $1,400 (Radio Santa Fe) to $200 (Radio Mundial), with an average cost per station of roughly $700. Monthly costs for stations in other cities varied directly with the size of the city: $700 in Medellin, $300 in Barranquilla, and an average cost of $225 for Cucuta, Pasto, Sogamoso, and Buenaventura (Table V-21).

Table V-21.   Estimated Cost per New Patient Added to Family Planning Programs through 1969 Radio Campaign, for Selected Clinics

	New Patients Added through Radio Campaign	Total Months of Radio Announcements during campaign	Estimated Average Cost of Radio Campaign	Estimated Total Cost of Radio Campaign	Estimated Average Cost per Patient Added
Centro Piloto (Bogota)	6,939	48	$700	$33,600	$4.80
Medellin	1,276	26	$700	$18,200	$14.30
Atlantico (Barranquilla)	371	28	$300	$ 8,400	$22.60
Cucuta, Pasto, Sogamoso, and Buenaventura (average)	—	15	$225	$ 3,400	—

[a]   New patients added through radio equal the net gain above projected new patients (see Table V-19).

[b]   One month of radio announcements equals one radio station carrying twenty announcements daily for a period of one month. Since announcements were generally carried over several stations for the period of the campaign, total months of radio in each city is equal to the sum of the months provided by each station.

[c]   Based on figures from Epoca Advertising, Inc., showing the monthly price for twenty 30-second announcements daily on each of the stations on which announcements were carried. Figures have been rounded to the closest $25.

In the three large city clinics (Centro Piloto, Medellin, and Atlantico) where the campaign clearly produced results, the estimated costs per new patient added are generally modest, at least compared with the range of costs estimated for the pamphlet and home visit approaches. While the absolute cost of the radio campaign in Bogota seemed high ($33,600), the cost per new patient attracted was very low ($4.80). The absolute cost in Medellin was much lower ($18,200), but the cost per patient ($14.30) was much higher. Of the three large cities, Barranquilla spent the least in total but the cost per patient in this city was $22.60. While little was spent on the radio campaign in the small cities of Cucuta, Pasto, Sogamoso, and Buenaventura, what was spent may have been wasted in terms of attracting new patients. The expenditure in these smaller cities may also have been less efficient in increasing public awareness—relatively large proportions of women in Cucuta did not recall the radio announcement and were ignorant of the term family planning. In conclusion, the campaign was most effective and most efficient in the larger cities, especially in Bogota.

Summary and Conclusions

The radio campaign in Colombia had a major impact on public awareness. Since high proportions of all age and educational classes of urban Colombian women listen at least occasionally to the radio, it was no surprise to find that, after only four months of the radio campaign, more than two-thirds of the women in Cali had heard a family planning announcement. By the end of the eight-month campaign the proportion who had heard an announcement was most certainly even higher.

The announcements taught several things. Many women, especially the young women, learned for the first time that a family planning clinic was available in their city. While most better educated women knew that "family planning" concerns birth control and contraceptive practice, only those less educated women who had heard the radio announcements were likely to have an equally correct understanding of the term. It thus appears that the radio announcements provided some new information about family planning to the less educated women who were initially rather ignorant of the term. In this way, the radio campaign democratized the spread of information. Moreover, after four months of the radio campaign in Cali, women in the younger age groups showed the highest awareness of existing clinic facilities. This is important because young women, having fewer children at present and with many fertile years ahead, are potentially best able to take advantage of clinic facilities to limit their completed family size. The overall influence of the Colombian radio campaign on public awareness is most apparent when its greater impact on the less educated and the young are taken into account.

Not all credit for increasing levels of awareness in Cali should be attributed *directly* to the radio campaign. The survey data reveal that over the period of the campaign, many women had read about birth control and family planning in books or magazines and that many others had talked with friends and relatives about these topics. This emerging reading and discussion was partly a result of the gradual evolution of the family planning debate in Colombia. Nevertheless, greater awareness of clinic facilities, greater understanding of the term family planning, and a greater freedom to talk openly about birth control, all generated by the radio campaign, must have contributed substantially to the growing discourse. Collective ignorance (where women find themselves in a social vacuum regarding the thoughts and opinions of their friends and neighbors on some topic) is surely breaking down on the family planning issue, and this is due in part to the radio campaign.

The impact of the radio campaign on public awareness was mediated not only by radio-listening patterns but also by the general attitudes in the community. In comparing response to the campaign in Cali with response in two other Colombian cities, Armero (very small, moderately traditional) and Cucuta (larger than Armero, yet very traditional), radio-listening habits are found to be directly related to size of community. The proportion of women who listened occasionally or frequently to the radio was highest in Cali (the largest city) and lowest in Armero. In contrast, awareness of clinic facilities and understanding of the term family planning were directly related to overall patterns of traditional religious attitudes and values, such that awareness was highest in Cali and lowest in Cucuta. It would appear that radio announcements have the most impact on women who are most open to new ideas on family planning and other issues. Typically, these are the young and the better educated in the modern cities.

While the radio campaign had an important impact on public awareness, its overall impact on contraceptive practice was rather small. In great part this seems attributable to the shortness of the period under consideration—one would not expect any substantial changes in contraceptive practice to occur over a period of four months, especially given that the final decision to adopt birth control generally comes after a period of thought and discussion on the issue. For example, it was found that the patient load in the Centro Piloto clinic of Bogota more than doubled after the campaign began, yet the great majority of new patients attributed their decision to go the clinic to discussions with friends or relatives. Only a few spontaneously mentioned the influence of the radio announcements. When the women were directly asked about the radio announcements, however, it was discovered that a high proportion had indeed heard them. Thus, the influence of the radio campaign is generally indirect, operating through increased interpersonal discussion of birth control among close acquaintances.

While the radio campaign had very little influence on overall levels of contraceptive practice, it nevertheless had a major impact on clinic attendance, especially in the larger communities. In a large city only a very small upward shift in the proportion of women seeking clinic services can produce a dramatic increase in the absolute number of new clinic patients. The fact that the campaign had little influence on the inflow of new patients to clinics in smaller, more traditional communities undoubtedly reflects in part the collective ignorance that surrounds family planning in these communities.

In various nations there seems to be some tendency for new clinics to grow rapidly in the first year or so and then to experience gradual declines. [25] While the causes of this may be diverse, a similar pattern was noted for the longer-established clinics in Colombia. It is interesting to note that the established clinics in Colombia that had entered into this decline phase returned to higher levels of new patient intake soon after the radio campaign began. In these cases the radio campaign not only brought in large numbers of new patients, who were unexpected on the basis of previous trends, but the unit cost of attracting these new patients by radio was extremely low, especially in comparison with the estimated cost of other public education techniques like pamphlet mailing and home visits by a family planning worker. The study disclosed that, in the context of a radio campaign, pamphlets and home visits do not add significantly to awareness of or interest in clinic services. Yet even if pamphlets or home visits proved to be more effective, as they have in Taiwan, radio still appears to be a more economical way of attracting new clinic patients.

In conclusion, the findings of this study suggest the following observations.

1.   In the absence of information campaigns to promote public awareness of and interest in family planning, newly established clinics will at first grow rapidly as they absorb the "backlog" of women who have accumulated over time looking for this service. As time passes and this backlog is diminished, the number of new patients entering will decline toward the rate at which women "naturally" become interested in family planning in that society.

2.   A public information campaign may increase clinic attendance in the early phases of clinic expansion by attracting previously motivated women who are looking for a service and who will respond immediately to a clinic address. Since these women would go to a clinic anyway, perhaps a few months later, the net gain to the overall program through attracting these women is minimal.

3. In addition to attracting previously motivated women, however, a public information campaign can create a new demand for family planning services among non-practicing, previously unmotivated women by increasing awareness of clinic facilities, by providing new insight into the meaning and utility of "family planning," and by creating an open social climate for discussing the issue.

4. The principal impact of the radio campaign on clinic development in Colombia appears to be indirect. Women hear the announcements, then discuss the issue with friends and relatives, and finally, on the basis of personal advice and support, some women develop interest and commitment. Radio is particularly advantageous, then, for it reaches a high proportion of women in all social-economic and age categories, it seems no more impersonal than the delivery of a pamphlet or a brief visit by an unknown family planning worker, and the women who hear the announcement know that their friends and neighbors have also likely heard it and may be willing to talk about it.

5. The effectiveness of radio must be qualified by the fact that it seems to work rather well in modern urban centers yet very poorly in traditional settings. This suggests that an ambience of traditional values and ignorance may effectively prevent women from adopting new practices. However, before this conclusion is accepted, an attempt should be made to direct radio announcements toward the level of discourse that traditional women can understand and accept. This would include, among other things, more careful and explicit explanations of the meaning of "family planning," its advantages, its simplicity, and its utility in spacing births as well as controlling number of children.

6. Finally, in evaluating the impact of a mass media campaign, the immediate impact of the campaign on clinic attendance is an important consideration. But of greater importance is the emergent influence of the campaign on public awareness, interest, and discussion, for these factors will determine the long-term success of the program. Future campaigns in Colombia should be directed both toward clinic attendance and public awareness.

Chapter VI

Radio and Family Planning in the Dominican Republic

Anthony Marino

Division of Social and Behavioral Sciences,
Stockton State College, Pomona, New Jersey

Official government activity in family planning in the Dominican Republic began in February 1968 when President Joaquin Balaguer established the National Population and Family Council (NPFC) within the Ministry of Health and Social Welfare. The Council's role was to develop a program of family planning services within existing public health facilities. By December 1968, nine family planning clinics had initiated activity and by the end of 1970 a total of thirty-two clinics were operating under NPFC sponsorship in twenty-six cities throughout the Dominican Republic. In the first eighteen months of the program, almost 20,000 women received family planning services, representing approximately 6 percent of the total female population in the fertile ages resident in the twelve districts having clinics at that time.

While the NPFC is the official government agency involved in family planning, the Dominican Association for Family Welfare (DAFW) is a private organization with similar interests and is affiliated with the International Planned Parenthood Federation. In 1965 the DAFW opened the first family planning clinic in the country in the capital city of Santo Domingo. This clinic, along with a second opened in 1967, became part of the NPFC system when that agency was founded in 1968. The organizations cooperate closely, and the head of the DAFW is a member of the Executive Board of the government family planning agency. In general, the NPFC is responsible for clinic operations while the DAFW assists the government agency in training clinic personnel and disseminating information on family planning.

By the beginning of 1970 the organization of the family planning clinics had moved forward well enough for both agencies to devote more attention to program evaluation. Starting in the spring of 1970 and continuing to the end of the year, the NPFC conducted or sponsored a study of clinic drop-outs, a national male KAP (knowledge, attitude, and practice) survey and a two-city study of mailed informational materials on family planning. In addition, the NPFC and DAFW collaborated in the development of a multi-media educational program at the national level and sponsored jointly a study of the impact of a short-term radio campaign in two small cities. This chapter reports the findings of the latter effort.

Design

Two small cities were selected for the radio campaign, each having only one local radio station. One city received a "high intensity" treatment of thirty family planning announcements a day for one month, while the other city's station broadcast only ten messages daily over the same period. Interviews were collected both before and after the radio campaign to determine changes in awareness of the clinics and family planning in each of the two cities as a result of the program. Ten different announcements were prepared by the staff of the DAFW covering such themes as the relationship between family planning and mother's health, the socioeconomic well-being of the family, the responsibility of parents to foster only the number of children they can provide for adequately, etc. Thus these messages had a *motivational* content in that they aimed to persuade women to take advantage of family planning services as preparation for attaining socially desirable goals.

In addition, the announcements provided *information* to the audience. Two of them were dialogue between supposed *campesinos* conversing in lower class idiom about the meaning of family planning. One message stated family planning services were free, and all of the messages ended by encouraging women to visit their local family planning clinic, the address of which was given by the local announcer. Each spot announcement lasted approximately one minute.

The two cities selected for the study were Montecristi and San José de Ocoa. In 1970 Montecristi had approximately 8,250 residents and San José de Ocoa had 9,380. Montecristi is a provincial capital located on the Atlantic coast in the extreme northwestern corner of the country near the Haitian frontier. The United Fruit Company formerly operated banana plantations in the area but closed down its operations in the early 1960s. The rural region is now dependent on subsistence farming and goat raising, while the city of Montecristi has some salt mining but serves mainly as a commercial and administrative center for the province of the same name. In general, the Montecristi area is economically depressed, and the government has recently proposed sugar cultivation and tourist facilities to revive the region's economic structure.

In contrast, San José de Ocoa is located in a fertile but relatively isolated valley in Peravia province in the south central portion of the Dominican Republic. Its economy is based on the many agricultural products cultivated in the area, and the city serves as a marketing center for the valley. Santo Domingo lies across the mountains less than forty miles away, though by road the distance between the cities is doubled. The rural population in the district surrounding San José de Ocoa is approximately five times as large as that of Montecristi.

Both cities have family planning clinics that are located in public health hospitals. Montecristi's clinic opened in November 1968; the facility in San José de Ocoa began operating in May 1969. By the beginning of September 1970, the starting date of the radio campaign, 1,702 women had received family planning services in Montecristi's clinic while only 228 women had gone to the clinic in San José de Ocoa. In the first eight months of 1970 the monthly attendance rates in Montecristi's clinic were approximately five times greater than in San José de Ocoa. Indeed, relative to the population of its immediate surrounding area, Montecristi's clinic had the highest percentage of clinic acceptors in the country while San José de Ocoa had the lowest.

The study involved a simple "before-after" design. A team of eleven female interviewers, students at Santo Domingo's Pedro Henríquez Ureña National University, interviewed approximately two hundred women aged 15 - 49 years (age and sex were the only criteria for sample eligibility) in each city a week before the initiation of the radio campaign and two hundred *different* women aged 15 - 49 years in each city a week after the radio messages had been discontinued. The pre-campaign round of interviewing took place in late August 1970. The radio messages were broadcast throughout the month of September, and the post-campaign interviews were collected in early October.

For the survey, based on maps compiled for the recent census, each city was divided into two parts at the point of the central plaza, each half serving as the area for either the "before" or "after" round of interviewing. This was done with the aim of reducing "noise" generated by the first round of interviews from affecting the post-campaign respondents. Within each half of the city interviewers were assigned blocks randomly drawn and instructed to interview one female respondent between the ages of 15 - 49 years in each house in her designated area. If there were two eligible respondents, they were to interview the younger if the house address ended in an even number and the older if it ended in an odd number. If three or more women in a given household were eligible the interviewers were to vary the age of the respondent selected in each succeeding case. Some bias was introduced by this sampling procedure inasmuch as women who were more likely to be home during the day had a greater probability of being interviewed and such women were also more likely to display a higher intensity of radio listening. A total of 393, or approximately 23 percent of the eligible women, were interviewed in Montecristi while 412, or 21 percent of the eligible group, comprise the San José de Ocoa samples.

Table VI-1 presents background characteristics for each of the four samples. Within each city the pre- and post-campaign samples are closely matched, though Montecristi women display a somewhat

Table VI-1. Selected Characteristics of Pre- and Post-Campaign Samples in San José de Ocoa and Montecristi

	San José de Ocoa		Montecristi	
	Pre-campaign	Post-campaign	Pre-campaign	Post-campaign
Mean Age	29.3	29.0	29.4	30.6
Percent currently mated	72	68	70	67
Percent mothers	77	72	75	75
Mean number of living children per mother	4.5	4.4	4.4	4.2
Mean ideal number of children[a]	3.3	3.0	3.1	3.3
Percent who say ideal number of children is between 2 and 4	78	79	72	77
Percent Roman Catholic	96	92	92	93
Percent with 4 or fewer years of schooling completed	56	52	43	40
Number of cases	(204)	(208)	(201)	(193)

[a] Women stating non-numerical responses (e.g., "All that God sends") were removed from base. The percentage of such women in each sample respectively was 7, 4, 7 and 8. The question was: "If you were starting your family now and could have the number of children you wanted, how many children would be ideal for you?"

higher level of school attainment. In all samples the mean ideal family size is approximately lower than the mean number living children. This discrepancy between ideal and actual will become even more pronounced as additional children are born, suggesting the potential interest of these women in family planning.

Radio-Listening Patterns

An important variable in this study is the relative success of each local station in reaching its audience (Table VI-2). Combining both samples in each city, 74 percent of the women in San José de Ocoa and 80 percent in Montecristi had radios in their homes. Many of those that did not have a radio claimed they often listen to a friend's or neighbor's set. A larger proportion of Montecristi women, 79 percent, tuned in their local station on an average day compared to the 59 percent in San José de Ocoa who listened to that city's station. In addition, audience levels in Montecristi were generally higher throughout the broadcasting day, but at night 52 percent of the San José de Ocoa respondents listened to their station as opposed to 33 percent in Montecristi. Within each city the local audience does not vary by education, but the Montecristi station attracts a larger proportion of women with four years of schooling or less. This is important inasmuch as these women comprise the major target population for the family planning program.

Table VI-2. Selected Indicators of Radio-Listening Patterns in San José de Ocoa and Montecristi (in percent)

	San José de Ocoa	Montecristi
Have radio in the home	74	80
Listen to local station on an average day	59	79
Those with 4 or fewer years of education who listen to local station on an average day	61	78
Those who listen to local station in the:[a]		
morning	21	69
midday	12	27
afternoon	17	37
night	52	33

NOTE: Unless otherwise specified, all tables refer to women aged 15-49 years.

[a] Percentages do not add up to 100 because of multiple mentions. About one-fourth of the 412 respondents in San José de Ocoa were not asked this question.

The relative popularity of the Montecristi station clearly emerges in Tables VI-3 and VI-4. In San José de Ocoa the local station is less popular than Radio Guarachita (transmitting from Santo Domingo as do all other stations on the list), though when one or two other stations are included as ones regularly tuned in by the respondents in addition to the favorite station, the stations reverse positions. Conversely, the local station in Montecristi commands a huge lead in popularity; 62 percent stated it was their favorite station and 85 percent named it as one of the stations they regularly hear. Radio Mao, broadcasting from the city of Mao-Valverde, is second but only named by 7 percent as their favorite station, though by somewhat more, 43 percent, as one they regularly listen to.

Given both its lower clinic-acceptor rates and the finding that its local station had a much smaller audience, San José de Ocoa was selected for the high intensity program of thirty announcements a day; the Montecristi station was assigned ten daily announcements.

Table VI-3. **Favorite Radio Stations and Stations Listened to Regularly by San José de Ocoa Respondents (in percent)**

Radio Station	Favorite Station	Favorite Station or Listened to Regularly[a]
Ocoa (local station)	21.6	56
Guarachita	27.3	52
Comercial	17.9	39
HIZ	6.6	21
Santo Domingo	6.8	19
Voz del Tropico	2.3	15
HIJB	4.4	10
Cristal	1.7	6
Mil	1.0	4
Universal	1.0	4
All other stations mentioned[b]	5.5	16
Never listens to radio	3.9	—
Total	100.0	
Number of cases	(412)	

[a] In addition to being asked to name her favorite radio station, each respondent was asked to list two other stations she also listened to regularly. Some respondents did not name additional stations.

[b] A total of eleven other radio stations was named.

Table VI-4.   **Favorite Radio Stations and Stations Listened to Regularly by Montecristi Respondents (in percent)**

Radio Station	Favorite Station	Favorite Station or Listened to Regularly[a]
Montecristi (local station)	62.4	
Mao	6.8	43
Santa Cruz	5.2	28
Beler	3.4	25
Quisqueya	1.0	10
Santo Domingo	1.7	9
Onda del Yaque	2.3	9
Santiago	1.2	8
Dajabon	1.0	7
Comercial	2.9	5
All other stations mentioned[b]	10.9	35
Never listens to radio	2.0	—
Total	100.0	
Number of cases	(393)	

[a] In addition to being asked to name her favorite radio station, each respondent was asked to list two other stations she also listened to regularly. Some respondents did not name any additional stations.

[b] A total of eighteen other stations were named.

Unfortunately the variable of high versus low intensity of announcements was not adequately tested. Arrangements had been made to have Radio Mao broadcast eighteen family planning messages daily starting in late July (five weeks before the beginning of the radio campaign). It was assumed that few women in Montecristi listened to Radio Mao and that the broadcasts there would not interfere with the one described here. But since the Mao-Valverde station was found to be the second most popular in Montecristi, women there, in addition to the ten daily messages carried on their local station, were exposed to the eighteen announcements broadcast by Radio Mao. In effect, then, both San José de Ocoa and Montecristi received a high intensity radio campaign.

Pre-Campaign Knowledge of Clinic Facilities

Another important variable in this study is the level of knowledge

Table VI-5.   Selected Indicators of Family Planning Knowledge in Pre-Campaign Samples, by City

Question	Answer	Percent Response	
		San José de Ocoa	Montecristi
Do you know if there is a family planning clinic in this city? (If Yes) Where is it located?	Gave correct location	53	81
Do you think you have to pay in order to have them help you at the family planning clinic?	No	56	76
	Don't Know	34	21
	Yes	10	3
Do you think it is easy or hard to have them help you at the family planning clinic?	Easy	58	72
	Don't Know	38	22
	Hard	4	6
Number of cases		(204)	(201)

concerning family planning services prior to the radio campaign. Ideally, pre-campaign levels of knowledge in both cities would be identical and any post-campaign differences between the two cities could be attributed to the differential impact of the radio campaign. But as shown by Table VI-5, there were significant differences in knowledge prior to the campaign, and knowledge in both communities was surprisingly high. In Montecristi 81 percent gave the correct clinic location versus 53 percent in San José de Ocoa.

Furthermore, Montecristi women were more likely to know family planning services were free and to perceive these services as easy to obtain. In order to assess the relative success of the campaign, an accounting should be made of the significant differences in level of knowledge before its initiation.

At the time the first round of interviewing was undertaken the Montecristi clinic had been operating for twenty-two months and San José de Ocoa's clinic for fifteen months. Thus, Montecristi women had had a longer opportunity to find out about their clinic. On the other hand, from the very beginning the number of new acceptors of family planning was much higher in Montecristi, and this trend persisted until the time of the study. One factor that may account for this is that although the population of the San José de Ocoa district is much larger than that of Montecristi's, the latter clinic actually does draw from neighboring communities, since it was until recently the only clinic in the northwestern region of the Dominican Republic.

Additional factors that may account for the differences in level of knowledge may be the relative quality of each clinic, the success of respective local efforts to inform women of the clinic's existence, and differences in the motivational disposition of women to practice family planning. Concerning the latter, no information is available that might lead to the conclusion that Montecristi women were more interested in family planning. As to the relative quality of each clinic, respondents who knew someone who had gone to the clinic were asked if they were satisfied with the service. In San José de Ocoa 92 percent and in Montecristi 89 percent said their friends were satisfied, showing no significant discontent with either clinic's services. It should be added that 40 percent in San José de Ocoa and 61 percent in Montecristi claimed they knew someone who had gone to the clinic, thus reflecting the higher clinic attendance in the latter city and the resulting feedback of this attendance into greater clinic knowledge in general in Montecristi.

This feedback is suggested by national clinic records, which show that approximately seven out of ten women who go to a family planning clinic cite a friend or relative as their source of information. It is well to note, however, that women may forget the initial source of clinic information, particularly if it is an impersonal one such as the radio or newspaper, in favor of naming the latest or most salient source for them at the time of the interview. This is demonstrated in Table VI-6, which shows how women in the samples learned of the clinics.

The proportion who mentioned radio before the campaign is quite low but rises to the most frequently mentioned source in Montecristi and the second most important source in San José de Ocoa after the radio campaign. Thus, in addition to indicating that the campaign had success in both cities, Table VI-6 also suggests that women tend to name the most recent salient source rather than the first, since the number of women who know about the clinic after the campaign is less than the number of women naming radio as their source of information, particularly in Montecristi. In short, it can be assumed that some of the women in post-campaign samples who cited radio as the source by which they found out about the clinic actually knew about it before the campaign.

Two other features of Table VI-6 merit attention. First, while most clinic acceptors in the nation as a whole name a friend or relative as their source of information, in the samples these personal sources of information are much less important. Hence, the decision to go to the clinic may involve a process of first finding out about it through a less personal source (radio, doctor, etc.) and then speaking about the clinic with a friend or relative who has already attended. If so, then the importance of adequately attending patients in the clinic is paramount, for they are probably the most effective means by which interested women are persuaded to go to the clinic.

The second point brought out by Table VI-6 is the high number of Montecristi women who cite an "other" source of information. When asked what it was, the majority stated "the sign over the hospital." They were referring to the words FAMILY PLANNING CLINIC painted in large red letters over one of the entrances to the hospital. The sign is difficult to miss by anyone entering the hospital compound and is even quite visible from the street. Since Montecristi is a small city and the hospital is near the center of town, most residents have probably seen the sign. Conversely, the hospital in San José de Ocoa is on the outskirts of the city and its clinic signs are small and confined to the interior of the building.

Table VI-6.   Source by Which Women Found Out about the Family Planning Clinic, by City and Sample

| | San José de Ocoa | | Montecristi | |
	Pre-Campaign	Post-Campaign	Pre-Campaign	Post-Campaign
Friend or neighbor	33	13	29	17
Relative	9	10	9	4
Doctor or nurse	43	35	28	21
Radio	2	32	1	37
Other	13	10	33	21
Total	100	100	100	100
Number of cases	(110)	(159)	(160)	(174)

NOTE: The question was: "Do you know if there is a family planning clinic in this city?" If yes, "How did you find out about the clinic?"

Impact of the Radio Campaign: Survey Results

Five factors must be considered in judging the relative success of each town's radio campaign: 1) the more favorable radio-listening patterns of Montecristi; 2) the higher level of education in that city; 3) the greater clinic acceptor rates in Montecristi; 4) the higher level of pre-campaign clinic knowledge in Montecristi; and 5) the higher number of announcements broadcast by the local San José de Ocoa station but offset by the family planning messages carried by another station that reaches Montecristi. By at least one indicator, both campaigns had some success (Table VI-6). A comparison of the proportion of women who claimed to have heard radio announcements before and after the campaign also points to the success of the campaigns (Table VI-7).

The question was asked, "Have you heard recently any announcements about family planning on the radio? How often?" Replies were categorized as "often," "occasionally," or "never." The first two categories have been combined. Three important points can be made about Table VI-7. First, within all four samples better educated women claimed to have heard announcements about family planning in greater proportions than did women with four years or less schooling. Second, within the same educational group, Montecristi women claimed to have heard the announcements more often than San José de Ocoa women. Third, after the campaign a much higher proportion of women in each educational group and in each city said they heard the messages than did women prior to the campaign. For the aggregate post-campaign sample, there is a change of percent of 49 and 53 in San José de Ocoa and Montecristi, respectively.

Table VI-7. Percent Who Heard Family Planning Messages on Radio, by Sample, City, and Education (in percent)

	San José de Ocoa			Montecristi		
	0-4 Years of School	5+ Years of School	All Women	0-4 Years of School	5+ Years of School	All Women
Pre-campaign	19	27	23	29	42	36
Post-campaign	62	82	72	82	93	89
Number of Cases						
Pre-campaign	(114)	(90)	(204)	(86)	(115)	(201)
Post-campaign	(109)	(99)	(208)	(77)	(116)	(193)

Even before the campaign, however, about one-fourth of the San José de Ocoa and one-third of the Montecristi women claimed they had heard family planning announcements on radio. Does this indicate a high level of response bias or did these women actually hear such announcements? The local Montecristi station had never carried specially prepared family planning announcements before, but women there listen to Radio Mao and this station started broadcasting announcements about five weeks prior to the first round of interviewing. Thus a number of Montecristi women may have heard radio messages concerning family planning without having been given any information on their particular clinic, since the Radio Mao announcements only mentioned the facility in Mao-Valverde.

On the other hand, the San José de Ocoa station had played one of the regular messages on family planning sporadically from about late 1969. However, no records were kept of when and how often it was broadcast. In addition, some of the Santo Domingo stations had carried panel discussions and some regular spot announcements on family planning throughout 1969 and early 1970. In both cities, therefore, women could have heard something about family planning on the radio before the local campaign.

Included in the interview were questions concerning three commercial products advertised on radio along with the fabricated names of three non-existent products. Over 90 percent of the respondents in both cities claimed they had heard announcements for the three well-known and heavily advertised products, while 13 to 28 percent stated they had heard announcements for the fictitious products of Calabria Spaghetti, Rio Verde Soda, and Marino Soap Detergent (Table VI-8). Clearly the number of women claiming to have heard announcements for products that do not exist is high enough to cause some concern. Moreover, women who stated they heard family planning messages were more likely to claim they also heard about both the real and false products than were women who did not hear the family planning announcements. But especially for the false products the difference between those who claimed to have heard and those who did not is not so large and, indeed, is reversed in Montecristi after the campaign. In addition, hearing announcements on all the items mentioned, including family planning, is also associated with frequency of radio listening. Women who listened to radio more frequently heard announcements for real items and thus perhaps honestly thought they must have also heard about the non-existent products. Nonetheless, given the response bias on this type of question, the number of women who truly heard radio announcements for family planning can be assumed to be somewhat less in all four samples than the percent recorded by the survey.

As noted, hearing family planning messages on radio is associated positively both with education and radio listening. Since the latter does not vary with education both seem to have an independent effect on hearing announcements. An important question, however, is whether or not higher frequency of listening to the local station can reduce or cancel the education relationship with hearing announcements in the post-campaign samples. Table VI-9 shows that this does occur in Montecristi, where the educational differential virtually disappears among women who listen to their local station on an average day, but not in San José de Ocoa. There both education and radio listening maintain a clear positive relationship with hearing family planning announcements. Conversely, in Montecristi it is only less educated women who do not listen to their local sta-

Table VI-8. Percent Who Heard Selected Products Advertised on Radio, by City, Sample, and Exposure to Family Planning Messages on Radio

| | San José de Ocoa | | | | | Montecristi | | | | |
| | Pre-Campaign | | Post-Campaign | | All Women | Pre-Campaign | | Post-Campaign | | All Women |
	Heard Message	Did Not Hear	Heard Message	Did Not Hear		Heard Message	Did Not Hear	Heard Message	Did Not Hear	
Products (Possible)										
Montecarlo Cigarettes	100	87	100	83	93	97	91	98	82	95
Bermundez Rum	96	87	97	85	91	100	95	97	86	96
Criolla Beer	96	86	97	83	91	98	91	94	82	94
Products (Impossible)										
Calabria Spaghetti	27	15	28	24	21	21	22	22	23	22
Rio Verde Soda	19	14	17	12	15	21	15	15	18	16
Marino Soap Detergent	17	6	18	10	13	19	13	13	14	14
Number of Cases	(47)	(157)	(149)	(59)	(412)	(73)	(128)	(171)	(22)	(394)

tion on an average day who are notably dissimilar to all other women in not hearing the family planning announcements.

These data help explain why the aggregate Montecristi post-campaign sample heard family planning announcements in higher proportions than in San José de Ocoa (89 versus 72 percent), since Montecristi women are both better educated and listen more frequently to their local station than women in San José de Ocoa. Thus the question arises as to what percentage of women in San José de Ocoa would have heard the announcements if they had had the same education and radio listening distribution as the Montecristi sample. By standardizing on the latter sample and multiplying by the actual percent of San José de Ocoa women who claimed they

Table VI-9. **Percent of Post-Campaign Sample Who Heard Family Planning Messages on Radio, by City, Listening Frequency, and Education**

	Doesn't Listen to Local Station on an Average Day	Listens to Local Station Less Than 2 Hours a Day	Listens to Local Station 2 or More Hours a Day	Total
San José de Ocoa				
0-4 years of school	45	67	78	62
More than 4 years of school	61	88	100	82
All women	53	76	89	72
Number of cases				
0-4 years of school	(38)	(39)	(32)	(109)
More than 4 years of school	(36)	(33)	(30)	(99)
All women	(74)	(72)	(62)	(208)
Montecristi				
0-4 years of school	33	83	96	82
More than 4 years of school	90	85	100	93
All women	73	84	98	89
Number of cases				
0-4 years of school	(15)	(18)	(44)	(77)
More than 4 years of school	(20)	(33)	(63)	(116)
All women	(35)	(51)	(107)	(193)

heard the announcements, approximately 82 percent, instead of the recorded 72 percent, would have heard the family planning messages in San José de Ocoa. The remaining difference between cities probably reflects the greater sensitivity to family planning that existed in Montecristi prior to the campaign, thus the higher proportion of women there who claimed to have heard the announcements.

Knowledge of Clinic Facilities

As a result of the large number of women who heard the family planning announcements, knowledge about the clinic could be expected to rise after the campaign. This is indeed the case (Table VI-10). In every cell but one there is an increase between samples. However, the change is slight on the question of payment for family planning services. One of the ten announcements did mention that the clinic was free but the message seems to have had no impact. Both perception of the ease of obtaining clinic services and the ability to name correctly the location of the clinic rise more noticeably. This increase is generally similar for both educational groups in each city. The radio campaign was unable to narrow the educational difference between women concerning knowledge about the clin-

Table VI-10. Selected Indicators of Family Planning Clinic Knowledge by Sample, City, and Education (in percent)

	San José de Ocoa			Montecristi		
	0-4 Years of School	5+ Years of School	All Women	0-4 Years of School	5+ Years of School	All Women
Correctly named location of the clinic						
Pre-campaign	46	62	53	73	87	81
Post-campaign	66	84	75	79	98	91
Think one does not pay to be helped in the clinic						
Pre-campaign	49	64	56	67	83	76
Post-campaign	54	66	60	65	86	78
Think it is easy to receive help in the clinic						
Pre-campaign	52	67	58	69	75	72
Post-campaign	65	75	70	74	85	81

NOTE: See Table VI-5 for the questions.

ic. But it did have success in narrowing the gap in knowledge between the two cities, particularly with reference to the location of the clinic. In San José de Ocoa the number of women who could correctly name the location of the clinic increases from 53 to 75 percent while in Montecristi it goes from 81 to 91 percent. But despite this significant rise in knowledge in San José de Ocoa, it does not exceed the pre-campaign levels of knowledge in Montecristi.

Returning to the consistent educational differential, it might be hypothesized that among women who said they heard the announcements the gap would be narrower than that for the aggregate sample. Table VI-11 shows that the 18 percentage point difference between educational groups for all women in San José de Ocoa does narrow to 12 points for women who claimed they heard the announcements. In Montecristi it drops from 19 to 12 percentage points.

Knowledge of the clinic's location is also slightly related to urban birth in Montecristi and to income in both cities in post-campaign samples. When education is controlled, however, these differentials all but vanish. Women aged 20 — 39 years were most likely to know

Table VI-11. Percent of Post-Campaign Sample Who Named Correct Location of the Clinic, by City, Education, and Exposure to Family Planning Announcements on Radio

	Heard Announcement	Did Not Hear Announcement	All Women
San José de Ocoa			
0-4 years of school	78	46	66
More than 4 years of school	90	56	84
Number of cases			
0-4 years of school	(68)	(41)	(109)
More than 4 years of school	(81)	(18)	(99)
Montecristi			
0-4 years of school	87	43	79
More than 4 years of school	99	71[a]	98
Number of cases			
0-4 years of school	(63)	(14)	(77)
More than 4 years of school	(109)	(7)	(116)

[a] Less than ten cases.

the clinic's location prior to the radio campaign, but age is related to both parity and education. In this study childless women and currently unmated mothers were included for the same reason they are normally excluded from others, namely, they are the least "sensitive" to family planning. The intent was to determine if the radio campaign could reach such women (Table VI-12).

Looking first at pre-campaign samples, childless women, as expected, were least likely to know the clinic's location, but once again the educational and city differences are the more important variables. Within each city, however, better educated women who have one to four children were most likely to know the clinic's location. Parity displays an uneven relationship with knowledge of the clinic by education. Among better educated women lower parity mothers were more acquainted with the clinic's location, while the opposite was true among less educated women. Perhaps among better educated women those who have the most children are more likely truly to want that number than are less educated women with the same parity. Hence their relatively lower interest in the clinic

Table VI-12.   Percent Who Named Correct Location of the Clinic, by Sample, Education, City, and Number of Living Children

| | San José de Ocoa | | | | Montecristi | | | |
| | Number of Living Children | | | | Number of Living Children | | | |
	0	1-4	5	All Women	0	1-4	5	All Women
Pre-campaign								
0-4 years of school	28	48	50	46	50	68	86	73
More than 4 years of school	41	77	61	62	84	90	83	87
All women	36	63	53	53	74	83	85	81
Post-campaign								
0-4 years of school	67	59	73	66	73	79	86	79
More than 4 years of school	88	82	90	84	100	98	100	98
All women	80	67	78	75	94	89	91	91
Number of cases								
Pre-campaign								
0-4 years of school	(18)	(40)	(56)		(16)	(28)	(42)	
More than 4 years of school	(29)	(43)	(18)		(37)	(60)	(18)	
Post-campaign								
0-4 years of school	(21)	(44)	(44)		(11)	(28)	(37)	
More than 4 years of school	(40)	(38)	(21)		(40)	(56)	(20)	

than might otherwise be expected looking only at education.

In general, the pre-campaign sample data suggest that women who know most about the clinic are those who have more reason to be interested in family planning, once the effect of education is controlled. But what is the case after the radio campaign? Within each parity group in Table VI-12 knowledge of the clinic's location increases, but the increase is greatest among childless women. Indeed, knowledge among this group is now higher than for both groups of mothers. Childless women are younger and better educated and also tend slightly to listen more frequently to radio. In short, this provides evidence that radio may be an excellent medium to convey family planning information to younger women who otherwise have limited personal sources of knowledge on the subject.

Ability to Explain Family Planning

Since family planning is a more socially acceptable though not entirely equivalent term for birth control, it should not be assumed that all women know what it means. This is not a moot point; the program in the Dominican Republic relies on the ability of women to understand that a family planning clinic is where one is provided with the means by which she can control her fertility.

The respondents were asked, "Have you heard about family planning? How often?" If the respondent answered "often" or "occasionally," she was then asked, "What does family planning mean? Can you explain it to me?" The respondent was given no hints and had to express the concept in her own words. The interviewers were instructed to probe at least twice (without giving any clues) before indicating that a respondent could not give a definition of family planning. Thus there are three categories of women: those who had never heard about family planning, those who claimed they had heard of it but could not define it, and women who could explain it correctly.

This method probably understates the true number of women who understood that family planning means controlling family size, since some, particularly the less educated women, may not have been articulate enough or were too embarassed to explain it. Whatever the case, considering only those who were able to correctly define family planning, Table VI-13 indicates that they are better educated, and that Montecristi women exceed their counterparts in San José de Ocoa. Again, the level of knowledge achieved in the latter city following the campaign falls short of Montecristi's level *before* the campaign. Furthermore, the educational differential among wo-

Table VI-13. Percent Who Could Correctly Define Family Planning, by City, Sample, and Education

	San José de Ocoa		All	Montecristi		All
	Years of Schooling		Women	Years of Schooling		Women
	0-4	5+		0-4 Years	5+	
Pre-campaign	47	68	56	61	86	75
Post-campaign	52	81	66	71	92	83

men widens considerably in San José de Ocoa while it narrows slightly in Montecristi after the campaign.

Impact of the Radio Campaign: Clinic Records

While survey data are helpful in assessing the radio campaign program, the most meaningful measure of success would be an increase in new patients at the family planning clinic. Monthly admissions records collected from each clinic by the central office of the National Population and Family Council were examined to this end.

There are, however, many problems in using clinic attendance data to measure real trends. For example, successful clinics have relatively fewer eligible women in the population as months pass compared to less successful clinics. Moreover, as new clinics are opened, older clinics continually face additional reductions in their eligible "constituency." Monthly clinic rates are also affected by political events (such as the Dominican presidential election of 1970) or by long holidays such as Christmas when clinics are closed. Hence December is normally a poor month and January a good one as the previous month's backlog of cases enters the clinic. Keeping these factors in mind, the average monthly admission rates for the fourteen family planning clinics that were opened prior to July 1969 are presented in Table VI-14. The first two columns show the average monthly new acceptors for the periods July—December 1969 and January—June 1970. The third column is the average monthly new acceptors for June—August 1970, and the fourth column presents the same data for the post-radio-campaign period of September to November. Finally, column five shows the percent change in monthly new acceptors between the September—November and June—August period of 1970. Attendance for December 1970 has been eliminated because of the generally lower rates resulting from the Christmas holidays.

Table VI-14. Average Monthly New Family Planning Acceptors for Selected Clinics and Time Periods

Clinic[a] and Total 1970 Population of Its District	Average Monthly New Acceptors				Percent Change between Columns 3 & 4
	(1) July-Dec. 1969	(2) Jan.-June 1970	(3) June-Aug. 1970	(4) Sept.-Nov. 1970	
San José de Ocoa (47,800)	13	14	10	21	+110
Mao-Valverde (43,300)	18	23	29	46	+ 59
Barahona (58,600)	93	54	39	56	+ 44
Montecristi (15,100)	76	63	63	84	+ 33
Puerto Plata (74,500)	77	70	78	84	+ 8
Santo Domingo (3 clinics, 817,500)	578	514	557	576	+ 3
San Pedro de Macoris (70,100)	45	43	39	39	0
Santiago (244,800)	209	183	216	200	- 7
La Romana (42,600)	25	36	42	37	-12
San Francisco de Macoris (126,300)	50	92	105	93	-11
Monción (7,600)	8	9	13	11	-16
Luperon (30,100)	27	23	28	22	-21

[a] The eighteen clinics opened in the Dominican Republic between July 1969 and December 1970 are not included in this list.

By presenting a six-month average the first two columns of Table VI-14 reduce the effect of a one- or two-month fluctuation. In three cities (Barahona, Santo Domingo, and Santiago) there was an appreciable decline in average monthly acceptors in the January—June 1970 period compared to the previous six months. This drop in clinic attenders was a by-product of the turmoil associated with the presidential election campaign in those three major cities. In gener-

Table VI-15. Percent of New Acceptors Who Found Out about
Family Planning Clinic through Radio, by Selected
Clinics and Time Periods

Clinic	June-August 1970	Sept.-Nov. 1970
San José de Ocoa	3	40
Mao-Valverde[a]	1	26
Barahona	0	0
Montecristi	1	19
Puerto Plata	0	1
Santo Domingo (3 clinics)	1	1
San Pedro de Macoris	0	10
Santiago	1	2
La Romana	4	4
San Francisco de Macoris	4	9
Monción	0	0
Luperon	0	1

NOTE: Each new acceptor was asked a series of questions on her first visit
to the clinic including how she found out about it.
[a] The first period in Mao-Valverde corresponds to May-July because the radio
campaign began there in late July.

al, other areas of the country were not as adversely influenced by
events surrounding the election proceedings. Moreover, Santiago's
clinic decline was also affected by the opening of a second clinic in
that city in the second half of 1969.

In June — August 1970, rates were therefore in part influenced by
the generally lower monthly averages of the preceding period. Thus
the increase in new acceptors registered by eight of the twelve cities
on the list in this period reflects the resumption of political normal-
cy, and, in turn, the September— November rates generally decline
or only slightly rise compared to the previous three-month period in
part because that period had higher rates than normal due to the in-
flux of women who had postponed their visit to the clinic until after
the election. In addition, many new clinics were opened in 1970,
and women who may in the past have made a long journey to an
older clinic were able to go to a closer one.

But the first four clinics on the list show a marked increase in new
family planning acceptors in the final three-month period. In effect,

all four are special cases. Barahona's clinic in the first eight months of 1970 was adversely affected by problems in maintaining a full clinic staff. (A Peace Corps volunteer working in the clinic was temporarily transferred to another city until after the election, and a shortage of medical personnel forced the clinic to operate at much less than capacity and to discontinue IUD insertions altogether for a few months.) Hence the 44 percent rise in new acceptors in the September—November period still left that clinic's rate of new acceptors far below the July—December 1969 average.

The other three clinics at the top of the list are also special cases because of the radio campaign in those cities. The monthly average of new acceptors more than doubles in San José de Ocoa, rises by almost 60 percent in Mao-Valverde, and increases by one-third in Montecristi. In San José de Ocoa and Montecristi this increase counters a previous leveling off trend while in Mao-Valverde there is a noticeable acceleration in the number of new acceptors in the post-campaign period. It may be concluded then that the radio campaign significantly boosted attendance in the immediate post-campaign period.

An alternative explanation might be that the rise in attendance was the result of the interview, which conveyed a pro-family planning message to the respondents. In San José de Ocoa, for example, where over 400 women were interviewed, if only 5 percent of the respondents went to the clinic, more than 60 percent of the increase in clinic attendance would be explained.

Two pieces of evidence can be cited to meet this objection. First, the increase in new acceptors occurred not only in Montecristi and San José de Ocoa where interviewing took place, but also in Mao-Valverde where no interviewing was done. Thus this latter city serves as an effective control case in this study. Moreover, as shown in Table VI-15, the proportion of new family planning acceptors who named radio as the means by which they found out about the clinic is markedly higher in the three locations where a radio campaign took place compared to other cities during the same period, and the proportion of new acceptors is also higher relative to the pre-campaign period in the same cities.

Conclusions

Based on survey findings and clinic records several important points can be made. First, the radio campaign was successful in each of the three cities where it was carried out. Clinic records demonstrate

that all three cities experienced a significant increase in new acceptors immediately after the campaign. The fact that this percentage
increase is highest in San José de Ocoa does not prove the program
was most successful there. Since its monthly acceptance rates were
previously quite low, any rise in the number of new acceptors produces a high rate of growth. On the other hand perhaps the lower
rates of the San José de Ocoa clinic reflected a population less motivated for family planning, and thus the large increase is testimony
to the campaign's impact. Whatever the case, if only the numerical
excess over previous monthly attendance figures is considered, then
Montecristi had the most successful campaign since it had the highest number of unexpected new acceptors relative to its district's population base. Parenthetically, the 2,042 women who had accepted
family planning services in Montecristi's clinic by the end of 1970 represent an astounding 117 percent of that city's female population
aged 15 - 49 years, 64 percent of the district's corresponding population, and 14 percent of all women aged 15 - 49 years in the province. Perhaps both an analysis of that clinic's records and an intensive study of the region's women with regard to their fertility attitudes and communications channels would be quite useful.

The radio campaign was also successful in creating awareness of
the clinic's location, in increasing perception that it is easy to receive
attention at the clinic, and in increasing ability to define family planning. The gap in knowledge between cities narrows after the radio
campaign but the educational differentials among women in each
city generally do not. Finally, there was evidence that radio may be
an effective information channel for younger women and for childless women.

Awareness of family planning and the clinic was relatively high in
each city, but particularly in Montecristi, even before the radio campaign. Most likely the relatively small size of these cities, where
word of the clinic does not have far to travel, explains much of this
awareness. But since a majority of women already knew about the
clinic they could be expected to be sensitized toward hearing family
planning announcements on the radio. This is suggested by the fact
that after accounting for both their higher average education and
frequency of radio listening, Montecristi women were more likely
than San José de Ocoa women to have heard the announcements, as
were better educated women in both cities.

Nonetheless, some women in all three cities were apparently persuaded to go to the clinic as a result of the radio campaign. This
could be a short-term effect, and clinic acceptance rates may return

to previous levels as time passes. Enough information has been gathered, however, to support continued use of radio in the Dominican Republic as one means of successfully informing and motivating women to practice family planning.

Notes

Chapter II

1. The International Population Program research team consisted of J. Mayone Stycos, Alan Keller, and Alan Simmons. Keller directed the project in the field.

2. Few neighborhoods in the city are truly homogeneous, and the neighborhoods in which clinics are located generally also contain substantial numbers of poor families.

3. In actual practice, the physicians more often play an active part in patients' selection of method. Moreover, patients often are unable to receive the official education program before seeing the doctor. Some never receive more than a brief introduction to the subject by the doctor; others may receive the doctor's favorite method with no explanation.

4. The varieties of oral contraceptives in use were Eugynon, Eugynon CD, Gynovlar, Ovulen, Ovulen 28, Ovral, Lindiol, and Riglovis. The IUD was the Lippes Loop, and the injection was the three-month variety of Acetate of Medroxiprogesterona.

5. R. Benitez, "Niveles Generales de Fecundidad en la Ciudad de Mexico Comparados con los de Otras Ciudades y Paises" (Paper distributed at the Latin American Regional Conference on Demography, Mexico City, August 1969).

6. M. Mateos Fournier, *Evaluación del Problema del Aborto Criminal en Mexico* (Mexico, D.F.: Fundación para Estudios de la Población, 1969).

7. Such percentages are in accord with those reported by J. Mayone Stycos for a more representative sample of Mexico City. J. Mayone Stycos, "Contraception and Catholicism in Latin America," *The Journal of Social Issues*, October 1967.

8. Robert G. Potter, "The Multiple Decrement Life Table as an Approach to the Measurement of Use, Effectiveness and Demographic Effectiveness of Contraception," in *A Handbook for Service Statistics in Family Planning Programs* (New York: The Population Council, 1968).

9. C. Tietze, "Modern Methods of Birth Control: An Evaluation," in *Family Planning Programs: An International Study,* ed. B. Berelson, (New York: Basic Books, 1969); M. Hall and W. Reinke, "Factors Influencing Contraception Continuation Rates: The Oral and Intrauterine Methods," *Demography,* 1969; J. Speidel and L. Weiner, "Continuance of Family Planning in a Health Department Clinic" (Paper available from Research Division, Office of Population, Bureau of Technical Assistance, U.S. Department of State, A.I.D., Washington, D.C., 1968). Tietze reports method continuance rates (not the same as clinic continuance) for the U.S. of 73 per 100 at one year for oral and IUD and 62 and 67 per 100 for oral and IUD respectively at two years. Hall and Reinke report method continuance rates of 48 and 59 for oral and IUD respectively at one year for Baltimore clinic patients. Speidel and Weiner discuss a *clinic* continuance rate in New York City of 60 at twelve months for oral patients. Additionally, Hall and Reinke report studies showing method continuance rates varying for the oral contraceptive from 8 in Turkey to 85 in England at one year, with the majority of studies between 50 and 80, and for the IUD from 69 in Taiwan to 85 in India. Much of the variance in these rates may be attributed, as Hall and Reinke emphasize, to varying definitions of termination of use and to differing follow-up procedures. What should be observed is that the *clinic* desertion rates in the FEPAC system are similar to *method* desertion rates reported for some other systems; thus, in sum, it would appear that the desertion rates in the FEPAC system are quite in line with those found in other programs.

10. These rates refer to women who had employed only one method. Rates were also calculated to include among users of each method the approximate 11 percent who had changed methods. Rates with "change" cases included did not differ for oral and IUD patients but did differ for the injection patients because of the higher percentages of women changing to the injection (about 33 percent of all injection users). As the relatively low attrition rate for "change" patients (regardless of the nature of the change) implies, women who change method quite probably are more motivated and perhaps better informed than other patients; thus the inclusion of a high percentage of such women among injection users did not afford an accurate picture of what desertion levels might be expected with the injection among more typical patients (the 89 percent who do not change method). It was therefore decided to utilize the tables excluding the method changers. A change in method was only so considered if it involved changing from one method group (IUD, pill, injection) to another. A change from one dosage of pill to another, then, was not coded as a change of method.

11.　The interview was initially developed in New York by Keller, Stycos, and Simmons and later refined in Mexico by Keller, Aurora Rabago, and Lic. José Morelos.

12.　The total percentage located varies by clinic from 51 to 67.

13.　At least 10 percent of the interviews conducted by each interviewer were repeated by a supervisor. Correspondence of replies was quite high, and no evidence of falsified interviews was uncovered. Later tests revealed little interviewer bias but did show that several interviewers were less able than others to elicit any sort of reply to several questions.

14.　These rates reflect experience with large populations and include both method and human failure.

15.　Method refers to most recent method. Approximately 11 percent of the women in the sample had changed methods one or more times.

16.　All women recorded as IUD users *after* desertion reported that they still had the IUD from the clinic. When levels of natural expulsion of IUD's are considered, it is reasonable to believe that most women are correct in their opinions.

17.　If the patient received advice from a doctor but supplies from a pharmacy, she was counted under the "doctor in hospital" category.

18.　Pill and injection patients, after the first visit and with the exception of occasional checkups, typically are seen more rapidly by the social worker or nurse.

19.　Side effects have also been reported by Tietze, *op. cit.*, and Speidel and Weiner, *op. cit.*, as the most frequently offered reason for discontinuance of use of oral contraceptives. Percentages of women giving this reason vary from 7 to 61.

20.　Reuben Hill, J. Mayone Stycos, and K. Back, *The Family and Population Control* (Chapel Hill: University of North Carolina Press, 1959).

21.　Stycos, *op. cit.*

22.　It may be, of course, that some women who deny having received the advice actually did receive it but did not absorb the "message."

23.　Age and education were found to have no relationship to knowledge, indicating a probable overriding effect of the clinic education program.

24.　A study by Leñero showed that 45 percent of predominately urban, adult Mexican respondents knew of no contraceptive method. Likewise Candano reported that 37 percent of Mexico City women living in an area similar to those inhabited by the respondents of the present study were unaware of contraceptive techniques. See L. Leñero, *Investigaciones de la Familia en Mexico* (Mexico, D.F.: Grafica Panamericana, 1968) and M. Mateos Candano, *Actitud y Anticoncepción* (Mexico, D.F.: Centro de Estudios de Reproducción, 1968).

25. The percentages were calculated using all respondents for three reasons. First, the relative order between clinics is unchanged on any variable from calculations using only deserters. Second, the use of the attenders tempers somewhat the more extreme view of the incidence of given factors yielded by an all-deserter sample and gives a more accurate view of the incidence of factors among *all* patients of a clinic. (Since 87 percent of the interviewees are deserters, however, the percentages still most strongly reflect the situation encountered among deserters.) Third, the active patient interviewees comprise approximately the same percentage of deserter interviewees in each clinic, and consequently no important bias is introduced by including them.

26. Within the sampling limits set—women living very far away were excluded from the study.

Chapter III

1. The team was directed by Parker G. Marden and J. Mayone Stycos, with field supervision by Axel I. Mundigo. Team members were Joseph H. Enright, Pierre Gauthier, Elsie Jackson, and Charles Teller.

2. The interviewing was done during the rainy season that followed a particularly severe drought. The importance placed on problems of inadequate water supply and, conversely, on the poor condition of streets and poor sanitation (both aggravated by heavy rain) may have influenced the results.

3. See Lisa R. Peattie, *View from the Barrio* (Ann Arbor: University of Michigan Press, 1968), especially chaps. 7 and 8.

4. Comments of these long-time residents about their lack of neighborliness are instructive: "My friends have all left the barrio"; "Those *meson* dwellers are here today, gone tomorrow"; and "We do not have real friends here, we just chat together in passing."

5. On the other hand, direct mass communications campaigns may be less effective in rural areas where the system of communications is not as well developed as in urban areas. Rural cultural patterns also may be more responsive to the more indirect method.

6. There were 844 children 0 — 9 years of age recorded in the interviews with Sample A, 25 percent of the total.

7. The only comparison that can be made between the 1961 Census of Honduras and the 1968 sample survey is for a ten-block area where the child-woman ratio rose from 709 in 1961 to 882 in 1968. This increase would seem to be due in part to changes in infant mortality and in part to actual increases in fertility.

8. The sex ratios for the ten-block area that could be compared were almost identical in the 1961 census and the 1968 sample enumeration. They were 114.3 and 115.9, respectively.

9. The ten-block comparison of change between 1961 and 1968 suggests that this underreporting may have occurred in both situations, despite differences in interviewers and procedures.

10. The ratio, therefore, is appropriately restricted to the child-bearing population (women 15 — 44 years of age). The influence of differences in age composition between populations that one might want to compare is minimal. Its few shortcomings are minimal and beyond the purposes of this paper.

11. If it were exactly 2.0, then the population would be declining gradually because of slight differences in the sex ratio at birth (more males) and the mortality of women before they complete their reproductive period.

12. United Nations, *Population Bulletin* (New York: United Nations, 1965), p. 66.

13. Naturally, the membership of each group is not permanently defined. The women in each category were placed there because of their marital status at the time of the study. By becoming married (or having children), women could move in one direction. By ending their union, they could move in the other. But, while the membership of the groups may change, their size and compositions will most likely remain relatively constant.

14. In Sample B, 21 percent of the respondents who did work for money worked less than ten hours, and 13 percent worked between ten and nineteen hours per week. Only 13 percent worked forty hours or more per week. The results are not directly comparable to those from Sample A because working housewives are disproportionately represented in the former sample, but they do suggest the amount of underemployment in the barrio.

15. From the pregnancy histories collected from women in subsamples A_1 and A_2, the infant mortality rate has been estimated to be approximately 150 deaths per 1,000 live births, and the foetal mortality rate at about 130 per 1,000 live births.

16.   The results of a study carried out in cooperation with the Departments of Preventive Medicine and Parasitology of the Medical School, Autonomous National University of Honduras, are instructive in this regard. Laboratory analysis of fecal specimens obtained from respondents in subsamples A_1 and A_2 revealed that 72 percent of the 401 persons studied had parasites, and 40 percent of these had two or more.

17.   The average number of children desired by males and females was $3.0 - 3.2$. See section on the communications campaign for elaboration and discussion.

18.   When one considers that the time period was only the preceding year, and that a number of families may have escaped major health problems during that period, this is truly a startling figure.

19.   The existence of a sizable minority who boil their drinking water, dispose of waste properly, and follow other sound health practices again suggests that there are several different "target" groups in the barrio.

20.   The Las Crucitas Health Center is designed primarily to provide maternal and child health services to a major part of the population of Tegucigalpa-Comayaguela. Major illnesses and injuries are treated principally at the San Felipe Hospital or other hospitals in the capital.

21.   These data require careful assessment. When respondents were asked specific questions of fact or knowledge (e.g., "When did you last use the Las Crucitas Health Center?" or "What services are provided at the Health Center?"), the answers can be viewed with confidence. But when the question required some evaluation of health services by the respondent, the results may be understated. Criticism is difficult to express to a stranger in any interview situation, especially in areas where evaluative comments are not made lightly. It is even more difficult when there is a clear difference in social status between the respondent and the interviewer, as was unavoidable in this study. The fact that many interviews were conducted by *gringos,* even though they all spoke Spanish fluently, or Honduran nurses (representing the very services that the respondents were asked to assess) made this situation even more complicated. But criticism was forthcoming. In Sample A, for example, more than 10 percent of those interviewed *spontaneously* criticized some aspect of the health services available to them. Given the interview situation, it would seem appropriate to treat unfavorable evaluative comments as understatements, although the degree to which they are understated is impossible to estimate.

22.   The researcher, a native Spanish-speaker, is a nurse with considerable background in health education and administration.

23. It should be noted, however, that the key phrase in describing the condition regarding health service is "delivery." Criticism of *the quality* of medical services provided by the staff of the Health Center was not intended. Detailed assessments of quality of care and the organization of health services in Honduras are beyond the scope of this report; nevertheless, it can be said that the quality seemed to present no major problems in the area of family planning, but the organization clearly did. Both topics warrant future scrutiny.

24. Some of the respondents offering spontaneous criticisms mentioned more than one reason. The most frequent combination was poor treatment and long waits for attention or crowded conditions.

25. At the time of the researcher's study, the results of the interviews had not been tabulated and were without influence. No attempt was made to focus upon the specific problem areas that persons interviewed mentioned.

26. Throughout this section the "after" sample will be used on the assumption that relationships with age and education will approximate those of the "before" sample.

27. The Disney film *Family Planning* and the Chilean *Una Mujer, Dos Destinos* were used.

28. Before the campaign, there had been some sound-truck and radio advertising on other health programs. In the "before" interview, 8 percent reported hearing both the sound truck and the radio, and an additional 23 percent the radio only.

29. Pills receive more emphasis in the clinics, especially in San Felipe. In 1968, 57 percent of Las Crucitas and 75 percent of San Felipe new patients received pills.

30. The estimate of the new cases is conservative, based on the official record of the clinic. The researchers counted about 13 percent more first admissions than appear in the official statistics.

31. Even in Las Crucitas the image of better service at San Felipe was apparent before the campaign. When asked whether they would prefer to go to Las Crucitas or San Felipe for family planning, despite its distance, almost as many chose the latter as the former. When asked the reason for their preferences, the large majority of those who chose Las Crucitas cited its convenient location rather than its service, while those who chose San Felipe almost invariably mentioned its superior services.

32. A higher proportion of the outsiders (69 percent) than insiders (54 percent) reported that they had heard about the clinic on the radio.

Chapter V

1. For a brief history of the organization of family planning programs in Colombia, see Thomas G. Sanders, "Family Planning in Colombia," *Fieldstaff Reports*, American Universities Fieldstaff, West Coast South America Series, vol. 17, no. 3 (Colombia, 1970).

2. Current crude birth rate in Colombia is estimated to be in the range of 41 to 44 per 1,000, and the crude death rate is estimated to be in the range of 12 to 14 per 1,000, yielding an annual growth rate for the year 1969 of approximately 3.2 percent. Dorothy Nortman, *Population and Family Planning Programs: A Factbook*, Reports on Population/Family Planning, no. 2, (New York: The Population Council and the International Institute for the Study of Human Reproduction, Columbia University, July 1970), table 4.

3. This figure includes only those PROFAMILIA clinics that were open to the general public. It excludes PROFAMILIA clinics in National Institute of Social Security hospitals (established in late 1969 and early 1970), which provide services to women covered by social security who have recently borne a child in one of these hospitals. This post-partum family planning program is important in its own right and is discussed briefly later.

4. Noteworthy in this regard is the volume *Población y Programas de Planificación Familiar* (Bogota: ASCOFAME and Tercer Mundo, 1967), containing articles originally published in English in *Population and Family Planning Programs*, eds. D. Bogue et. al., (Chicago: University of Chicago Press, 1965).

5. An important collection of ASCOFAME articles on knowledge, attitudes, and practice of family planning among professional groups and the public in Colombia appeared as *Regulación de la Fecundidad* (Bogota: ASCOFAME and Tercer Mundo, 1968), vols. 1 and 2.

6. For example, Albert Lleras Camargo, twice president of Colombia, noted in Washington on July 9, 1965, that the way to stop the population explosion was "through demographic control." In the same year Carlos Lleras Restrepo, a politician, economist, and future (1966 - 1970) president of Colombia, said that Colombia could not avoid a demographic policy. Sanders, *op. cit.* p. 3.

7. Given that detailed summaries of the activities of the ASCOFAME-administered program are confidential, the author is limited to crude estimates based on limited information. The number of clinics involved in the program and the number of these currently reporting some activity were provided by ASCOFAME. To estimate the number of new patients in each clinic in a given period, however, forced reliance upon personal impres-

sions gained through visits to several of these clinics over the period from 1967 to 1969. The estimates produced therefore must be interpreted very cautiously indeed.

8.   These data are based on a breakdown of new patients by type of contraceptive method chosen for the first quarter of 1970, made available by PROFAMILIA.

9.   However some anomalies are apparent. The two Barranquilla clinics combined have attracted fewer women proportionately than has either the Bucaramanga or the Cucuta clinic, despite the fact that the latter were not established until 1968. The Medellin clinic, established in 1966, also seems to have accomplished relatively little. While there is no factual explanation for the low results in Medellin or Barranquilla, Colombian folklore suggests two possible answers. Medellin is the capital of the department of Antioquia, which is generally regarded as one of the most conservative areas of the country and has been long noted for its strong family ties and high fertility. Barranquilla, a principal Atlantic port of Colombia, is dominated by a distinctive Caribbean culture with a predominately Negro and Mulatto population characterized by high rates of consensual unions and illegitimacy. A small proportion of the eligible population that Cali seems to have attracted clearly reflects the short span of time for which the clinic there has been operating.

10.   Information on the growth of the Mexico City clinics was kindly provided by Dr. Alan Keller of the Fundación para Estudios de la Población (Mexico).

11.   The author is especially indebted to Mrs. Elsie Jackson for a descriptive account of several PROFAMILIA clinics in operation. Mrs. Jackson, a nurse with considerable experience in family planning programs in the U.S. and Puerto Rico, visited PROFAMILIA clinics in Cartagena and Bogota, spending some time in each clinic observing and chatting with patients and staff.

12.   All women were selected from a sample frame developed as part of a nationwide fertility sample survey carried out by ASCOFAME in July and August of 1969. The Bogota sample was chosen by distributing the population according to block, and choosing a random sample of city blocks so that large blocks had a proportionately greater possibility of being selected. One hundred and fourteen blocks were chosen, half of which were of upper and middle class status. Approximately two thousand women residents in these city blocks were enumerated to determine age, marital status, education, and number of living children. From these, five hundred to six hundred women were selected for ASCOFAME interviews.

From the enumeration list 881 women were chosen aged 15 — 44 with at least one child, living in the lower and middle class areas. These women were then distributed randomly into three experimental groups, of roughly equal size. To estimate the percent who were infertile, the percent already attending a family planning clinic, and those otherwise ineligible to respond to communication and go to PROFAMILIA, the women visited at home (the visit group) were interviewed briefly on these topics at the time of the family planning worker's contact. Information from the interview by the family planning worker and from the previous basic census by ASCO-FAME allows an assessment of the probable demand for contraceptive services and determination of some of the characteristics of the eligible population.

13.   The reasons for non-response included: not present in the house despite several visits, out of town, deceased, and indirect refusals of various kinds. Indirect refusals occurred primarily in the middle strata and help account for the high non-response rate (23 percent) in this group. The indirect refusals generally took the form of repeated postponements of the interview or of forcing the interviewer to talk with the maid at the door and never letting her enter and speak with the woman of the house. Many of the middle class women refused to speak to the family planning workers claiming that they already knew all they needed to know about birth control. (This study confirmed that 60 percent of the middle class were using or had used some form of birth control as opposed to 40 percent for the population as a whole.)

14.   Ronald Freedman and John Y. Takeshita, *Family Planning in Taiwan* (Princeton: Princeton University Press, 1969), chap. 3.

15.   Reuben Hill, J. Mayone Stycos, and K. Back, *Family and Fertility in Puerto Rico* (Chapel Hill: University of North Carolina Press, 1959).

16.   M. Beal and J.M. Bohlen, "The Adoption and Diffusion of Ideas in Agriculture" in *Mass Communication and Motivation for Birth Control,* ed. D. Bogue (Chicago: Community and Family Study Center, University of Chicago, 1967), pp. 78-81.

17.   For a review of these studies see Florangel Z. Rosario, "An Analysis of Social-Psychological and Cultural Variables Found in Family Planning Studies" (Ph.D. diss., Syracuse University, 1970). See especially the chapter Sources of Information.

18.   A report on newspaper coverage of the birth control and family planning controversy in Colombia for the year 1967 may be found in J. Mayone Stycos, "Colombia Tackles Her Population Problems," mimeographed (Ithaca, N.Y.: International Population Program, Cornell University, 1967).

19.   These announcements were written and distributed for broadcast by the advertising agency Propoganda EPOCA Limitada, Bogota.

20.   The Population Division of ASCOFAME, with the technical collaboration of the United Nations Demographic Center (CELADE) in Santiago, Chile, has recently (1970) completed a series of surveys in rural and urban areas throughout Colombia to estimate baseline levels of current fertility, family planning communication, and abortion in each region. The author is indebted to the Population Division of ASCOFAME for permission to analyze and report findings from several questions on contraceptive practice and family planning communication from their survey of Cali in July 1969.

21.   The author wishes to acknowledge the collaboration and invaluable assistance of Dr. Ramiro Cardona, director of Socio-Demographic Studies, Population Division, ASCOFAME, and Mr. Frank Traina of the International Population Program, Cornell University, who worked together to construct the final interview schedule and coordinate its administration. The field work was capably supervised by Mr. Alvaro Perez of ASCOFAME.

22.   The June and September samples differ in several ways. The former selected women aged 15 - 49 years, regardless of marital status. A rather high proportion (29 percent) were women under age 20 who had never been mated and who had never borne a child. Conversely, most of those over 20 years of age had been mated or were mated and had borne at least one child. In contrast, the September survey included only ever-mated women aged 20 - 49, and was stratified by social status, such that a high proportion of women with more than five years schooling was included.

For the June survey, proportional samples of city blocks were taken in each of these strata; all women in the city blocks chosen were enumerated, and a random selection of women included in this census were interviewed. The September survey differed only with regard to the sampling within strata, for a larger than proportional number were sampled from the higher social strata.

23.   A frequent limitation of survey work stems from the tendency for respondents, particularly those among less educated groups in traditional settings, to answer affirmatively questions they do not fully understand or on which they do not have a strong opinion. This "yea-saying" response set is frequently attributed to a desire on the part of the respondent to please the interviewer. Since the interviewer is typically of higher status and a guest in the respondent's home, politeness may demand that he agree as often as possible with his guest. To estimate the magnitude of such a response set, the respondents were asked whether they had ever heard announcements promoting several other services and programs. Thus, in addition to asking about family planning, they were asked if they had ever heard announcements on vaccination programs, certain brands of soap, cooking oil, and

cigarettes. The list included both items that exist and are advertised in Colombia, and several fictitious items whose brand names were fabricated.

Response bias is indicated by the percent who claimed they had heard the fictitious announcements and is sufficiently high to give some concern (Table V-12). Between 5 and 15 percent claimed they had heard advertisements on these products. Perhaps since the Spanish names Tequendama and Zipa are both common in Colombia, more people reported hearing advertisements for the oil and soap products with these brand names than Green River Cigarettes (Cigarillos Rio Verde), a name that sounds strange in English or Spanish. While the proportion who claimed to have heard of these false products is rather similar for those who heard an announcement on family planning and those who did not, the proportion who had heard of any of the real products is substantially higher than those who heard the announcement on family planning. This supports the hypothesis that radio-listening patterns are the principal determinant of hearing the family planning announcements.

24. The June survey determined contraceptive practice by asking, for each of eleven common birth control methods, whether the women had ever heard of them or used them. Since practice was probed for each method and the implied definition of prior use included single trials, the survey indicated rather high levels of practice—57 percent of ever-mated women in Cali reported having tried a method at some time. The September survey, in contrast, simply asked women whether they had ever used a method and when they began practicing it. Lack of detailed probing by method and the implied definition of prior use as "practice over a period of time" (beginning at some specified period, etc.) yields a much lower estimate of use—39 percent of ever-mated women in Cali reported having used a method (Table V-16). While age-education patterns of use are similar for the June and September surveys, the great disparity in absolute levels of practice which the different interview procedures yielded makes it impossible to directly compare the two surveys.

25. See, for example, the comments on Ceylon, Hong Kong, South Korea, Taiwan, Tunisia, and Singapore by Bernard Berelson, *The Present State of Family Planning Programs*, Studies in Family Planning, no. 57 (New York: The Population Council, September 1970), pp. 1-11.